The baby challenge

For women with a physical disability, pregnancy and motherhood can present a daunting challenge. Often more disabling than the disability is the difficulty in obtaining the range of information, facilities, and support that other pregnant women can expect.

The Baby Challenge is a clear and informative handbook that fulfills this vital need. It suggests the practical ways in which a woman with any physical disability can best prepare herself for pregnancy and motherhood and shows how health professionals can best support her. By presenting a wealth of information and drawing on the personal experiences of large number of disabled mothers, the book addresses the crucial questions that concern women with a disability.

This handbook is a serious attempt to close the gulf of ignorance that all too often prevents disabled women from experiencing the best possible care and encouragement.

The Baby Challenge presents a positive and practical approach for women with a disability who are contemplating childbirth and also for everyone involved in providing antenatal and postnatal support. It will be invaluable to undergraduates, lecturers, and practitioners in midwifery, obstetrics, and general medicine.

The Author

Mukti Jain Campion is a television producer who has made a number of films about parenting with a disability. She is the mother of a young son and an active member of the Disability Working Groups of the Maternity Alliance and National Childbirth Trust which aim to improve the support available to disabled parents.

The baby challenge

A handbook on pregnancy for
women with a physical disability

First published 1990
by Routledge
11 New Fetter Lane, London EC4P 4EE

Simultaneously published in the USA and Canada
by Routledge
a division of Routledge, Chapman and Hall, Inc.
29 West 35th Street, New York, NY 10001

© 1990 Mukti Jain Campion

Typeset by LaserScript Limited, Mitcham, Surrey
Printed and bound in Great Britain by
Mackays of Chatham PLC, Chatham, Kent
British Library Cataloguing in Publication Data

Campion, Mukti Jain, *1960–*
    The baby challenge: a handbook on pregnancy for women with
    a physical disability.
    1. Physically handicapped women.   Pregnancy & childbirth
    I. Title
    618.2

Library of Congress Cataloging in Publication Data

Campion, Mukti Jain, 1960–
    The baby challenge: a handbook on pregnancy for women with a physical
    disability / Mukti Jain Campion ; foreword by Wendy Savage.
    p.   cm.
    Includes bibliographical references.
    1. Pregnancy in physically handicapped women.   2. Pregnancy,
    Complications of – Popular works.   I. Title.
    RG580.P48C36 1990
    618.3–dc20   89-39067
                                                           CIP

ISBN 0-415-04858-3
ISBN 0-415-04859-1 (pbk)

For
Isobel and Mark
who helped me to see

Contents

Contents

Foreword

Wendy Savage

It is a great pleasure to be asked to write a foreword for this important and much needed book.

In recent years, there has been an increase in the 'medicalisation' of pregnancy and childbirth, to the extent that some women feel they have to say to their carers, 'I'm not ill, I'm just pregnant.' This attitude is one with which the disabled have to live every day. For some disabled women, therefore, the thought of conceiving and bearing a child is made even more of a challenge because of the inherent doubts foisted upon them by society in general and the medical profession in particular. We are not geared to accept the disabled (try coping with a normal shopping precinct in a wheelchair); to accept a disabled woman's wish to be a mother is difficult for the able-bodied, who take such things for granted. Doctors and midwives are not taught to cater for the special needs of disabled pregnant women, who thus face more obstacles than usual when seeking help.

Now with the publication of *The Baby Challenge*, there is an opportunity for disabled women to face the 'challenge' with optimism and a wealth of practical advice. It provides encouragement for mothers-to-be with a wide range of handicaps; it also gives general practitioners, midwives, obstetricians, students and all those concerned with the care of pregnant women a comprehensive source of information and lists of organisations offering advice and support. It should be on the shelf of every surgery and antenatal clinic office, thus helping to change the received wisdom about both pregnancy and disability.

Ruth Cochrane MRCOG
Wendy Savage FRCOG

Acknowledgements

There are many people who have given of their time and knowledge to check the accuracy of the medical information contained in this book, and while any errors remain my responsibility, I would like to gratefully acknowledge their contribution.

The following have kindly helped with individual chapters in Part 2:

Dr Barbara Ansell, Northwick Park Hospital
Dr Tim Betts, Aston University
Professor Robert Dixon, St James's Hospital, Leeds
Dr H. Frankel and Sister Diane Cooper, Stoke Mandeville Hospital
David Howard, Royal Throat, Nose and Ear Hospital, London
Dr Simon Nightingale, Queen Elizabeth Hospital, Birmingham
Dr Judith Steel, Royal Infirmary, Edinburgh
Dr Michael de Swiet, Queen Charlotte's Hospital, London
Phill Watson, ASBAH

Many other professionals, such as midwives, health visitors and social workers, have painstakingly read the book in its various draft stages and I am particularly grateful to obstetric physiotherapists Marge Polden and Jill Mantle for their constructive criticisms. My sincere thanks also to Dr Ruth Cochrane (founder of *Womanschoice*) for casting an obstetrician's eye over the final typescript and for her encouraging support of the book thereafter.

My greatest appreciation must go to all the disabled mothers who took the time to fill in my questionnaires and talk to me about their own experiences of motherhood in the hope of helping other women in similar situations. I would also like to acknowledge the commendable work of Jo O'Farrell in England and Tali Conine, Elaine Carty, Faith Wood-Johnson, Mary Lau, and Judith Thiele in Canada in collating information on parenting and disability – their efforts have been of great help in writing this book.

And lastly, what writer can adequately acknowledge the forbearance and support of their partner? In my case, I am particularly grateful to my husband for sharing his medical knowledge and for helping me to make sense of many useful sources of medical information and to translate their jargon into comprehensible English – no mean feat!

Introduction

Over the past decade attitudes to childbirth have begun to change. Health professionals are starting to recognise the importance of actively involving prospective parents in decisions about how we have our babies. Antenatal classes encourage us to understand the process of childbirth and to prepare for a baby's arrival. There are literally hundreds of books for first-time mothers who want to understand what is happening to their bodies and how to make informed choices about where and how they may have their babies.

But there are thousands of women these books never address, who often do not have an equal opportunity to get information and choice. I was 5 months pregnant with my first child and working as the producer of a BBC television programme about disability when I first became aware of the dismal lack of information available to disabled women contemplating pregnancy.

I made a film with a mother who has cerebral palsy and who was going through her second pregnancy – the difference between the information and support to which she had access and what was available to me was appalling.

The film was transmitted and prompted many disabled viewers to write with their own experiences of childbirth. Again and again, I read comments such as, 'It felt like I was the first disabled woman ever to give birth. There was no information; even the professionals sometimes didn't seem to understand my disability. . . .'

Despite a recent census by the OPCS, there are still no figures describing the number of women of childbearing age who are affected by a physically disabling condition. Nor are there any detailed figures relating to the number of disabled people with dependent children. Even if these figures existed, they would not reveal the number of disabled women who have decided NOT to have children because of lack of information or support. My own estimates suggest there must be several tens of thousands of women in this country who have a disabling condition and who are of childbearing age.

I was curious to see what information and support does exist and also what else could be unearthed from otherwise inaccessible sources and made readily available. So I set about researching the factual information and also devised a questionnaire to send to women who had already experienced parenting with a disability. The response was huge and I am indebted to all those who filled in the questionnaire or talked to me about what had often been a very difficult time.

Women with physical disabilities obviously vary enormously in their degree of handicap and the reader may at first question the legitimacy of a single book that addresses itself to all women with a disability. My conclusion in researching the experiences of nearly 200 women has been that a large number of challenges may be the same, whatever the nature of the disability. These are:

1. Lack of accessible and accurate information which causes anxiety and precludes choice.
2. Access difficulties in buildings and due to inappropriate equipment such as high hospital beds, inadequate provision of adapted toilets and so on.
3. Feelings of isolation due to not meeting others in the same situation.
4. Lack of understanding support by health professionals who seem only concerned with the medical outcome.

All these problems are interrelated and all too often combine to undermine a disabled parent's self-esteem and confidence.

The single most important factor that disabled women share is a desire to be treated as normal. Pregnancy is a potentially hazardous process for any woman, able-bodied or not. Just like anyone else, the woman with a disability wants to be treated as an individual who may need some specialist help – not to be treated as helpless or peculiar.

This book is intended for every woman with a physical disability contemplating pregnancy and its purpose is to help make your pregnancy as trouble-free as possible by anticipating the problems you can do something about and preparing you to cope with the ones that you can't. It assumes you are a woman first and disabled second and that, given adequate information, you are capable of making responsible decisions about parenthood.

My aim has been to provide as much factual information as I could find as well as to share some disabled mothers' experiences of their own pregnancies. This book is not, of course, to be used in place of consulting your GP or specialist but should help you become as well-informed as any able-bodied woman.

I hope that professional carers such as doctors, health visitors and midwives will also read this book and feel better able to provide more insightful care as a result of understanding the worries and special needs of women with physical disabilities. The individual case histories could also provide a useful basis for discussion in a teaching environment.

Finally, a plea, particularly to health professionals – please help increase the information that is available in the future by documenting case histories in professional journals and elsewhere. There is not enough information available at present in many of the areas I have looked at. You can change that.

(If any reader has information or details of helpful organisations that should be included in future editions of this book, I would be happy to receive such correspondence c/o the publishers.)

Part one

First steps in deciding to start a family

If you are considering whether or not to have a child at a particular point in time, there are likely to be two major considerations, depending on the nature of your disability and the capability of you and your partner. These are the practical and medical feasibilities of having a child: will you cope with looking after the child and is there any risk to the child or to yourself because of your disability?

Since the majority of disabled women can have babies safely, if given appropriate care, let's look at the practical feasibility first.

Practical feasibility

Whether you will be able to cope with looking after a child is something that only you and your partner can ultimately decide, but here are some points worth discussing together. These are also points which a GP, health visitor or other professional can discuss with a woman or couple who approaches her for advice. There are no right or wrong answers but the discussion should help a couple assess the reality of looking after children and perhaps the right time to start a family. The final decision should always remain with the couple.

How well-adjusted do you think you are to your disability?

How active a life are you able to lead?

How much help do you require with daily tasks?

Is your disability likely to deteriorate in the future or result in a shorter life span? If so, is your partner able, and prepared, to take on the additional responsibilities of bringing up a child?

Do you have a network of friends and/or relatives nearby on whom you can call for support both emotional and practical?

Have you any experience of looking after other people's children?

Do you foresee any major practical problems with looking after a child?

Do you live in accommodation that is suitable, or can be adapted, for you to look after a child?

Do you have a garden for messy play? (It can be a real essential if you have difficulty in doing things on the floor or tidying up.)

Are you reasonably secure financially?

Do you live in a community, for example, a village or housing estate, where you are known and where you know other people with young children? If not, would you consider moving?

Do you feel you will be a burden to your children? Is this a real possibility or a guilty worry?

Do you have a good relationship with your partner and would he be supportive?

Do YOU have confidence in your own ability to face the challenges that come with looking after a growing child?

Is it fair on the child?

This worry was voiced by many of the disabled mothers I spoke to and by many of the health professionals too. Would the children be ostracised for having a mother that looked different and/or was unable to do some of the things other mothers do? And would the children miss out in any way?

To answer these questions it would be necessary to establish what it means to be a 'good parent', and no one would suggest that there is only one sort of good parent. Will it matter in the long term that you were not able to kick a football to your child? Or that you weren't able to run along a sunlit beach with him as in some perfect 'cornflakes packet' family advert? Surely what matters is the quality of the time that you spend together and what you do, rather than what you don't do. As with any potentially stressful situation, your disability can have a positive effect or a negative effect, depending on how you share it as a family.

I am not suggesting that all will be straightforward if only you handle it correctly, but it does seem to me that the problem rests largely with other people's lack of understanding, rather than on the disabled woman's decision to have a child.

Society's attitudes will not change unless disabled parents are seen to have the same spectrum of needs as able-bodied parents. There is a real need for more positive images of disabled parenting and for more research into the effects on children of disabled parents. Without this research, the negative image of children who become slaves caring for their disabled parents, is the most alarming one that predominates. This in turn affects the attitudes of health professionals and undermines the confidence of disabled parents, often preventing them from seeking help when it is needed.

There has been a little research in this area and it has shown that if you, your friends and relatives are positive about your disability, the child will learn to be so too. Before school, most children don't worry about any differences, but once they start to mix with other children, the differences may be pointed out and can be hurtful if you are not there to explain – that, for example, although there are some things you may not be able to do, there are others that make you special and possibly more accessible.

As long as the child does not doubt your ability to love him and you do not fall into the trap of trying to over-compensate all the time, the chances are that the child will grow up well-adjusted to your disability and probably more independent, resourceful and considerate than other children. Remember, too, that not all able-bodied people are 'perfect' parents. If people had to pass a test before being allowed to have children, I suspect a lot of able-bodied people would be deemed unsuitable parenting material.

As for the long-term effects on children with disabled parents, there is some research which shows again, that, if the parents are well-adjusted to their disability and well-supported by others, the children are no more likely to suffer than if their parents were able-bodied.

In teenage years children sometimes go through a difficult phase of rejecting their parents and, if the parents are disabled, they may blame the problems on the disability. Again, it is important to recognise that teenagers often go through such phases anyway, but if it becomes seriously disruptive, counselling from a family therapist, for example, can help. It may also help to talk to another family in a similar situation (the National Childbirth Trust (NCT) Contact Register might be a useful starting point for this).

At the time of writing, a major research project has been initiated by the National Children's Bureau to look at the effects of disability (positive and negative) on children of parents with Parkinson's disease. Among other things, it intends to look at the sources of support such families have and how readily accessible and appropriate they are. This will certainly be of great value as such information does not presently exist and is vital to understanding the real problems that face families where a parent is disabled in this way.

In Appendix B there are some references about child development in children whose parents are disabled.

The next step

You may, after this discussion, decide that parenthood is not for you at present. For some couples this decision is more painful than for others but it is important to come to it together. It may help to seek counselling from your GP or perhaps a RELATE (formerly called Marriage Guidance) counsellor.

If, however, you emerge from such a discussion feeling positive and confident, proceed to sorting out the medical feasibility. If you're fairly confident but not sure, why not talk to someone with your disability who has had children? One way to do this is to contact the various self-help groups (see specific disability chapters in Part 2 for addresses) and ask to be put in touch with someone in your area. Another approach is to contact the NCT Register for Disabled Parents and see if they can suggest anyone with your disability that you could talk to.

Medical feasibility

The chances are that you know your disability and capability better than anyone else but just need more information relating to how pregnancy and childbirth will affect you and whether your condition will affect the pregnancy and the unborn child. Talk through your concerns with your partner and prepare a list of things you want to know – write down everything that worries you, even if it seems trivial. It's better to ask than to have it niggling away and causing anxiety later on.

You need to determine the feasibility from a medical point of view of your ability to have a safe pregnancy and labour, and to bear a healthy child. Your doctor (GP or specialist) should provide medical facts related to your disability and pregnancy. Since he will be familiar with any medication you might be taking and their potential effect on the unborn child, these can be changed and eliminated as necessary. If the medication is necessary, the doctor can discuss the need to consider the risk to the child before making a decision.

Risk to the mother

The risk to you will depend on your disability and how healthy you are, so you will need information and planning appropriate to your individual situation. There are a few disabling conditions which make pregnancy dangerous (for example, cystic fibrosis) but not necessarily impossible. Preventive planning and good medical care can help eliminate many of the risks associated with specific disabling conditions, for example, urinary infection and constipation which may be dangerous to a woman with a spinal cord injury.

Risk to the child

With some disabilities (multiple sclerosis, for example) no added risk to the child has been found. In some disabilities there is a risk which can usually be controlled by early medical care and intervention (for example, tendency towards early labour in women with spinal cord injuries), but with some there is a considerable risk (systemic lupus erythematosus, for example) and pregnancy may be discouraged. However, every woman is different and your situation should be assessed individually.

Genetic counselling

You will either already know or your GP will be able to tell you whether there is any genetic origin to your disability. If there is a chance that there may be, he may refer you and your partner to a genetic counsellor. The counsellor educates parents-to-be on the risk of having a child with a birth defect or disease after carefully examining the medical history of the couple and their families. A good counsellor will give you an understanding of probability, paint a picture of what it would be like to have a child who is disabled, explain the genetic causes to allay feelings of guilt, and spell out the reproductive options open to you.

The final decision about parenting will always be left to you and your partner.

Table 1.1 Reproductive and contraceptive considerations for women with physical disabilities. (Adapted from *Family Planning Services for Disabled People*.)

Condition	Female Reproductive Implications	Female Contraceptive Implications		
		Diaphragm	IUD	Pills
Amputations	Menstruation, fertility unaffected except in hemicorporectomy	Assistance needed if upper extremities involved	Client unable to check strings if upper extremities involved	Contraindicated if vascular or circulatory problems occur
Blindness/Visual	Menstruation unaffected Pregnancy unaffected unless diabetes involved Genetic counselling may be indicated			May be contraindicated if impairment due to diabetes, glaucoma, or vascular disease
Cancer – Breast or Reproductive System	Fertility, menstruation may be affected depending on organs involved, related hormonal function and therapeutic measures used Pregnancy may represent increased risk		May be contraindicated if malignancy is uterine	Contraindicated if estrogen based
Cardiovascular Accident (CVA, Stroke)	Menstruation, fertility unaffected			Absolutely contraindicated; other options depend on dexterity
Cerebral Palsy (CP)	Menstruation, fertility unaffected	May be difficult for client to place	May be difficult to insert	May be contraindicated
Epilepsy, Migraine	Fertility, menstruation unaffected Pregnancy probably unaffected			May either cause conditions to become less manageable or improve them
Multiple Sclerosis (MS)	Menstruation, fertility unaffected Pregnancy possible, may or may not exacerbate MS symptoms (no		May be contraindicated because pelvic inflammatory disease	May be contraindicated

	conclusive study)		(PID) and other problems could remain undetected due to lack of sensation	
Muscular Diseases	Menstruation, fertility, pregnancy unaffected Genetic counselling essential for women who have dystrophies of genetic origin	May be difficult to insert if upper extremities involved	May be difficult to check strings if upper extremities involved	May increase the risk of thromboembolism
Polio	Fertility, menstruation unaffected Pregnancy and delivery may be difficult for women with back deformity		May be contraindicated due to increased anemia	
Rheumatoid Arthritis (RA)	Fertility, menstruation, pregnancy unaffected Pregnancy often responsible for remission of symptoms; symptoms (pain and swelling) often reoccur about six weeks postpartum	May be difficult to insert due to hand deformities	May be contraindicated	May be contraindicated
Scoliosis	Fertility, pregnancy unaffected Genetic counselling indicated	May be difficult to insert or fit	May be difficult to insert or fit	
Short	Fertility usually unaffected; Turner's syndrome includes infertility Pregnancy rarely carried to full term; Caesarean delivery usually indicated	May be difficult for a woman with extremely short arms	May be difficult to place properly	May be contraindicated
Spinal Cord Injury (SCI)	Menstruation, fertility unaffected Menstruation may be delayed up to one year following trauma Pregnancy carries increased risks (i.e., urinary infection, decubiti, autonomic hyperreflexia during labour and delivery)	May be contraindicated because PID and other problems could remain undetected due to lack of sensation	May be contraindicated because PID and other problems could remain undetected due to lack of sensation	May be contraindicated when circulatory problems are present; thrombophlebitis could go undetected due to lack of sensation in extremities

Source: US DHSS (1981) *Family Planning Services for Disabled People – a manual for service providers.*

For some conditions, such as spina bifida, Friedreich's Ataxia, muscular dystrophy and some forms of blindness and deafness, the genetic risk to the baby should be considered, and the GP will refer you to a genetic counsellor or your specialist may be able to advise you.

Whoever does advise you should be adept at communicating the nature of the risk and also understanding that where one or both parents have a disability, they may be less aghast at the possibility of having a mildly handicapped child than an able-bodied person might be. Also beware that statistics are in themselves not very useful: they have to be put in a context. Again, a good specialist or genetic counsellor would be able to do this.

If you decide after all these consultations to go ahead and start a family, take some time to prepare yourself first.

Your GP should be able to advise you about diet, avoiding stress and getting as fit as possible despite any disability. He can also check that you have been vaccinated against rubella (German measles) and that you have had a recent cervical smear test. If you need either of these, then it is important to get them done before you become pregnant. Your doctor can also arrange for pregnancy tests to be done when your period is two or more weeks late and will probably refer you to the hospital for your antenatal care if the tests are positive. At this stage you could discuss the various options available to you for your antenatal care and where you may have your baby (see next chapter).

Family planning

Your doctor may also help you to plan the best time for becoming pregnant by giving contraceptive advice. Not all contraceptives are safe for or easily utilised by some disabled women, so the doctor needs to be familiar with specific contraindications for each disability. For example, women with circulatory problems should not be given the combined Pill as a means of birth control (see Table 1.1).

If you intend to have more than one child you will probably think quite carefully about the intervals at which to space them. There are many things to take into account when making such a decision, but it is worth remembering that an older child who can understand and obey you and be fairly independent is much easier to cope with when you have a new baby. Also, if he is at playgroup or school you will have some time with the new baby and for yourself. There may be further considerations arising from your particular disability: for example, if it is one that is likely to deteriorate, in which case you may plan to have further children sooner rather than later, or not at all.

Sexual difficulties

If you can, talk to your GP or your specialist. It is unfortunate that most health professionals are not taught much about sexuality so the amount of help they can offer to individuals with problems may be very limited. For more specific help, the Association to aid the Sexual and Personal Relationships of People with a Disability, SPOD (a well-respected and long-established charitable organisation), provides personal counselling as well as a number of helpful leaflets. You can ring them or write to them, at the address given on page 13.

The organisation also holds study days for professionals such as midwives and doctors as well as for self-help societies that invite them to talk to groups of people with a particular disability.

Fertility problems

If you have difficulty in becoming pregnant your GP is unlikely to refer you for investigation before you have been trying for at least a year. There are few disabilities that actually impair fertility in a woman but you may be taking drugs that do have an effect on your menstrual cycle. Again, discuss this with your GP or specialist. There are some disabilities (for example, spina bifida, cystic fibrosis) that affect fertility or complete ejaculation in men, and obviously if your partner has one of these disabilities you should seek advice early on in your relationship.

I spoke to one of Britain's leading specialists in the treatment of infertility and asked him whether he would ever hesitate to offer treatment to a couple where one or both partners had a disability. He was quick to reply that he had no moral right to discriminate in this way, and that he would only hesitate in the rare instances where pregnancy or childbirth might threaten the woman's life because of her existing disability. He emphasised the need to look at each couple's individual situation before deciding on the best course of action.

The father's role

This book is about pregnancy and childbirth and focusses largely on the woman going through the experience. However, I hope the baby's father will also find it useful and will feel able to get involved in the whole process. My research in talking to many mothers with disabilities has suggested that fathers fall into three broad categories: those who play an active role in supporting the mother and caring for the child; those who take a benign interest and help occasionally; those who remain uninvolved and apparently uninterested.

Most fathers seem to fall into the first category and, because of the disability, are usually well experienced in working as a team with their partner and therefore well prepared for dealing with a new situation such as pregnancy and parenthood.

The third type of father is not necessarily beyond redemption but is often made to feel excluded and useless, so has no motivation to get involved. Health professionals should make a point of involving the father and respecting his right to information and support. A father who is involved right from the start is more likely to enjoy parenthood and to support his partner in a useful way.

Contacts:

National Childbirth Trust Register for Parents with Disabilities
Judy Vickery
13 Chelsham Rd
London SW4

The Association to aid the Sexual and Personal Relationships of People
with a Disability (SPOD)
286 Camden Rd
London N7 0BJ
Tel. 071-607 8851/2

Association of Sexual and Marital Therapists
P.O. Box 62
Sheffield S10 3TS

Further reading

Darnborough, A. (1988) *The Sex Directory*, Woodhead Faulkner.
A directory of contacts and literature for people with disabilities.

National Childbirth Trust (1984) *The Emotions and Experiences of Some Disabled Mothers*, National Childbirth Trust.

Duffy, Y. (1979) *All Things are Possible*, A.J.Garvin and Associates.
A personal look at the sexuality of disabled women.

Heslinga, K. (1974) *Not Made Of Stone*, Woodhead Faulkner.
A frank look at the practical aspects of sex for the disabled.

Bullard, D.G. and Knight, S.E. (1981) *Sexuality and Physical Disability – Personal Perspectives*, Mosby.

Comfort, A. (1982) *Sexual Consequences of Disability*, Stickley.
Contains a range of articles on sex and disability.

Stewart, W.F.R. (1979) *The Sexual Side of Handicap*, Woodhead Faulkner.
A clearly written book aimed at the caring professions.

The Task Force on Concerns of Physically Disabled Women (1978a) *Towards intimacy: Family Planning and sexual concerns of physically disabled women*, Human Sciences Press.

The Task Force on Concerns of Physically Disabled Women (1978b) *Within Reach: providing family planning services to physically disabled women*, Human Sciences Press.

US DHSS (1981) *Family Planning Services for Disabled People – a manual for service providers*, Washington, DC: US DHSS.

This may be of interest to professionals wanting to provide better care to the disabled in this country. It explains many of the myths and the reality about sexuality and disability: etiquette, communication, medical aspects of specific disabilities and so on. A very comprehensive reference book for all, even though it is aimed at American readers.

Howland, C. (1986) *The First Time Parents Survival Guide*, Thorson.

This does not mention disability but is a very entertaining and sensible appraisal of the negative as well as positive aspects of having a child.

Chapter two

Getting the best out of the support services

Your pregnancy will be medically supervised by your GP, the antenatal clinic (probably, but not necessarily, at a hospital) and, perhaps, your own particular specialist. A number of other professionals, notably midwives, will play a crucial role in your care, and between all these highly qualified and experienced people, the chances are that your medical care will be very good.

The main purpose of this book is to help ensure that the access you have to information and choice to enjoy the experience of childbirth is the same as for an able-bodied woman. Since many of the disabled mothers I spoke to were less than happy with this aspect of the care they received, I think it is worth taking a closer look at how you can get the best out of the system.

The general practitioner

Your GP is the starting point for most medical care you receive on the National Health Service, so it's worth being on good terms with him or her. The GP's skills lie in recognising the nature and seriousness of your medical problems and knowing when to refer you to specialists. He is also at an advantage in that he can get to know you and, perhaps, your family over a period of time and can therefore see your problems in more of a context than, say, your specialist who may see you only once or twice a year.

GPs are much criticised, partly I suspect, because their diagnostic and communicating skills need to be applied to such a wide variety of situations that they do not always succeed in satisfying everyone all the time. People's expectations of what a good GP should be also vary a lot – some people want him to take over responsibility for their health, others want to know all the facts and to share that responsibility. Some want a fixer (like a car mechanic), others want a good listener and ally against their illnesses.

Most GPs do not see that many disabled people who are not elderly, so their direct experience of disability may be surprisingly limited – but, remember, they should have access to more information and can call on specialists to advise on specific medical aspects of a disability. How much they take advantage of this access to specialists depends on the individual GP.

Problem GPs

Some GPs may seem to pose problems. The fact that they only see you when you are ill or need help may lead them to regard you as dependent and therefore question your ability to raise children. Some GPs, like any other cross-section of the professions, may be arrogant, patronising and unhelpful: if you feel you have one like that you should change as soon as possible.

If you feel that your GP is just a poor communicator and that he never gives you the information you want, you could improve the situation by coming better prepared to appointments with him and being persistent. If you don't understand something, ask him to explain it again, omitting any medical jargon as necessary. Make sure you understand and accept the reasoning for any treatment he prescribes – and then follow it through when you leave the surgery. If the advice he gives is impossible to follow because of your disability or your lifestyle, say so.

Choosing a GP

If you have just moved to a new area you can get a list of local GPs from the library. Work out the ones closest to you and the most easily accessible, then ask around for recommendations. If a woman doctor is important to you, then find a practice that has one. You can find out age, sex and qualifications by looking up the doctor's surname in the Medical Directory at the local library. Find out the surgery hours and see if they suit your lifestyle. When you have settled on two or three, go and visit them. Check the accessibility, friendliness of reception staff, and whether the doctor has room on his list for new patients.

A group practice may be a good idea (especially if it has a baby clinic and health visitor attached to it). You can get to know a number of GPs and try to see the one with whom you get on best. If you have had bad experiences with a GP in the past, don't assume they are all like that: be positive and remember that a good relationship requires a bit of effort on both sides.

If you would like to change GPs within the same area, it is possible but may be more difficult. Most doctors are likely to be suspicious as to why your relationship with your previous GP has broken down – you don't have to give a reason, but you may be asked. However, if the new GP you choose accepts you on to his list all you have to do is to send your medical card to the Family Practitioner Committee (address on your medical card or under F in the phone book) with a covering letter. The FPC arranges the transfer of your notes.

Antenatal medical care

Your disability is likely to mean that your pregnancy may need closer supervision than otherwise and it is therefore important to attend all your antenatal appointments even though you may feel perfectly well. Don't put off going to get medical care if you become pregnant. A few recently publicised stories of children being taken away from disabled parents for fostering, may have caused many prospective disabled parents to fear a similar outcome, should some health professional or social worker decide they are not 'fit' parents. This is highly unlikely to happen, particularly if there is an opportunity to minimise the risks to both you and the baby with good medical care and appropriate practical support before and after the baby is born.

Antenatal clinics

These clinics can take place in a variety of places: at the hospital where you will have the baby, your GP's surgery, or a midwives' unit. Once you are booked in you should attend the clinics regularly throughout your pregnancy. If you have any problems with access, notify the clinic early and see whether they can be solved (by using a different entrance, for example, or arranging special parking provisions).

If the hospital clinic is difficult to get to, you may be able to have some of your check-ups at your GP surgery ('Shared Care') or even at home by community midwives. Many women hate going to the antenatal (or 'anti-natal' as one of my correspondents inadvertently spelt it) clinics because of the long waits and the often impersonal treatment.

You CAN ask to see a specific doctor and the likelihood is that if your disability is such that your pregnancy needs special attention, you will probably be seen by a doctor rather than a midwife.

Your first appointment at the clinic will probably take place around 11 weeks into your pregnancy (that is, 11 weeks from your last period) or even earlier. This is the most thorough of the checkups. Your partner should try to attend this appointment with you and thereafter as often as he can manage. It will involve him in the whole process and give you both the opportunity to discuss any worries with the obstetrician.

A midwife or doctor will take your medical history, check your cervix and uterus, make a note of your blood pressure and weight, and take samples of urine and blood to check for various things including signs of diabetes and anaemia. He may also arrange for an ultrasound scan to check the age of the foetus and how it is developing (and also to check whether there is more than one!). All these checks are routine but important to all pregnant women.

You may then meet the consultant obstetrician (the most senior doctor in charge of pregnant women) who will look at your medical notes and discuss with you any potential problems due to your disability, and how to prevent or manage them. He may have information from your specialist and your GP but you should use this opportunity to ask him anything that is worrying you.

The obstetrician may be able to tell you at this stage whether he thinks you will be able to deliver your baby vaginally or whether you will need a Caesarean section. Make sure you understand the reasons he gives as this is a point that worried many of the mothers with whom I spoke. A Caesarean section is not without risk (albeit a small one) and does not guarantee a 'normal' child, so the decision to perform a Caesarean should not be undertaken without very good reason.

Not all women see the consultant obstetrician at their routine check-ups but if there is anything that concerns you, you can ask to make an appointment with him. For example, if you are concerned about whether or not it is safe for you to have an epidural in labour, he may arrange for one of the senior anaesthetists to come and have a chat with you.

After this first check-up you will probably have monthly appointments until 28 weeks when they will become more frequent. At these subsequent check-ups they will probably only take your weight, blood pressure and urine sample, feel the position of the baby and, later on, listen to his heartbeat. If you are unable to stand on the weighing scales, some hospitals have harnesses in which you can be supported.

They may also decide not to bother with regular weighing as long as your 'bump' continues to grow, and may give you regular ultrasound scans instead.

If at any point in between appointments you are concerned about the baby or your own health (for example, if you notice any bleeding at any stage), contact your GP or the hospital immediately. The chances are that all is well but it is best to have any symptoms investigated so that you are reassured. Remember, too, that your obstetrician can consult your specialist (for example, a neurologist or rheumatologist) at any stage during your pregnancy or labour for advice relating to your disability, and you are entitled to ask him to do so if there are any particular concerns.

If you experience any problems with the attitudes of any of the health professionals who are supposed to be caring for you, try to resolve them through discussion at the time. If this does not work, you are entitled to ask to see a different person at your next appointment. Don't grin and bear it – unless they understand what has happened, they cannot improve the care they provide to other women.

Tests

There are a number of tests that doctors can now use to check the health of your baby before he is born. Most women accept the obstetrician's decision to have such tests as he deems necessary. If you have any concerns about a test, do discuss them with the doctor or midwife – you do not have to have any test if you are not convinced of its necessity.

Ultrasound is now routinely used to chart the progress of the foetus within the womb and you will probably have at least one scan during your pregnancy. In early pregnancy, you will be asked to come to your appointment with a full bladder, to lie on your back and to uncover your tummy. Scans later on in pregnancy will not require a full bladder.

A gel is spread on your skin to help make contact with the plastic disc transducer that passes high frequency sound waves (you cannot hear them and they do not hurt) through your abdomen and uterine walls to 'bounce' off the baby and give a picture on the television screen beside you. This is a very exciting moment as you can actually see what your moving baby looks like as early as 8 weeks.

Sometimes the picture needs explaining because the baby may be in an odd position at that moment. Ultrasound scans give a lot of information. They can tell how many foetuses are present; size and development indicate their exact age in weeks; the functioning of the heart and kidneys can be observed and many abnormalities detected. They may show up other interesting things like fibroids in your womb. These are harmless, benign growths that tend to enlarge during pregnancy and then shrink again after the baby is born – they usually pose no problems, but some women find them painful.

There is no evidence that ultrasound is harmful in any way either to you or the foetus and thousands of scans are carried out on pregnant women each month, apparently without any ill-effect.

If your disability makes it difficult for you to lie on your back, it may still be possible to scan you on your side or propped up with cushions. The skill of the person interpreting the scan will be more challenged as other organs may get in the way of the womb and confuse the picture. Similarly, if it is difficult for you to come to the appointment with a full bladder, it may still be possible to do a scan, but the picture may not be as clear.

A new scanning device which uses the same ultrasound technique but in the vagina rather than over the tummy is now coming into use. Its great advantage is that it does not require the bladder to be full to give a good image early in pregnancy. It is no more complicated or uncomfortable than having a cervical smear test and will be of great use to women who have difficulty in coming to the scan with a full bladder, who have colostomy bags or who cannot lie flat on their back.

Alpha feto protein (AFP) test. This is a blood test normally carried out between the 16th and 18th week of pregnancy. A small amount of blood is taken from the arm to measure the levels of a certain protein called AFP. A high level of this protein indicates the possible presence of spina bifida.

However, this test is not conclusive in itself and further tests (amniocentesis and/or detailed ultrasound scans) are necessary to determine whether there is anything wrong with the baby.

Amniocentesis is a test usually carried out at 16 weeks to test for the presence of spina bifida and Down's Syndrome in the foetus. It is usually only offered to women over 35 or other women who are thought to have an increased risk of having a baby with one of these problems. There is a very slight risk associated with the test (less than 2 per cent) that you may miscarry or go into early labour.

The test does not take very long and can be done as an outpatient appointment. You will be asked to come to the appointment with a full bladder. To perform the test, a local anaesthetic is given to numb the abdominal area. A fine needle is then passed through your abdomen into the amniotic sac surrounding the foetus and a sample of the fluid it contains is removed. Ultrasound is used to locate the exact position of the foetus and the placenta so the needle can be accurately placed to avoid harming it. The sample is then sent away to be tested.

Amniocentesis can also detect other conditions such as Turner's Syndrome, some inherited metabolic disorders (such as Tay-Sachs disease) and certain sex-linked conditions.

If you would not consider terminating your pregnancy should you be told that you were to have a child with any of these conditions, then it is probably not worth having the test. However, if you are at risk, it may help put your mind at rest.

Chorionic villus sampling (CVS) is a fairly new technique for early detection of conditions that previously have not been detectable until 16 weeks of pregnancy by amniocentesis. It is not yet widely available and is only offered to women who are considered to have a greater risk of carrying a baby with an abnormality. CVS cannot detect the presence of a neural tube defect such as spina bifida.

If the CVS test is available, it will usually be carried out between the 8th and 11th week of pregnancy. The test involves doing an ultrasound scan to show the position of the placenta. A tiny portion of the chorionic tissue is then removed from this and sent off for testing. The removal of the tissue is done in one of two ways: by inserting a fine tube into the vagina and through the cervix or by passing a needle through the abdomen and into the uterus.

The test may be a little uncomfortable but should not cause pain. A general anaesthetic is not necessary. Mothers are recommended to rest for a while after the test and then to take things easy for a couple of days, particularly avoiding any heavy lifting or strenuous exercise.

Results are usually available in 4–14 days. The advantage of the test is that congenital abnormalities can be detected in the early part of pregnancy and abortion offered if the parents do not wish the pregnancy to continue. This may be of particular importance to women who already have had a child with such an abnormality.

A higher risk of miscarriage is associated with the CVS test than with amniocentesis, but, because it is a relatively new test and also because it is done early in pregnancy when the natural miscarriage rate is higher, it is difficult to know exactly what the miscarriage rate associated with CVS is.

X-rays are rarely used nowadays in early pregnancy because of the associated risk to the developing foetus. However, the risk is deemed smaller later in pregnancy when the baby is less vulnerable. The only reason X-rays may then be used is if there is a worry that the baby's head may be too big to pass through the mother's pelvis.

Maternity care

Maternity care varies depending on where you live. When you first become pregnant ask your GP about what help is available in your area and who you can expect to see during your pregnancy. Ideally, you should be visited at home at least once by both a health visitor and a midwife. In practice, staff shortages mean that you may only see one of these. The crucial thing to remember is that you can ASK to see any of the professionals for specific additional help or advice.

Midwife

A midwife is a professional who is trained to look after women going through a normal pregnancy, labour, and postnatal period, to recognise any deviation from the norm if it arises, and to refer a woman to the doctors if necessary. Midwives also run antenatal classes.

Most midwives work in maternity wards, but community midwives care for women at home too. Depending on where you live, you may be visited by a community midwife during your pregnancy. For women who are severely restricted in their mobility, community midwives may be able to do most of your antenatal checks at your own home. Again, ask about such provisions if they would help you.

The midwife can advise you on preparing yourself for the birth of your baby. You can discuss the style of labour you would like and also ask for ideas about labour positions. If your disability limits your movements, you may wish to know the options that you will have in labour so that you can try the positions out in advance.

Immediately after the baby is born and you are back home, a midwife will visit you at least once a day for a week or more, checking on your recovery and the well-being of the baby.

In some areas you may be able to get to know a team of, say, 4 midwives antenatally, one or other of whom will deliver your baby in hospital and, all being well, will return home and look after you from 6 to 12 hours after the birth. Usually only 'low-risk' mothers are allowed home so soon after birth and if this is your first child the alternative of having this so-called Domino delivery but staying in hospital for 2 to 3 days, is more realistic.

Home births

Many disabled women would prefer to give birth at home because the discomforts of being in an unfamiliar hospital environment add substantially to the problems of being a new mother. If your disability is one which does not put you or the baby at any additional risk during childbirth (for example a visual or hearing impairment), you may be able to persuade your GP – particularly if this is not your first child and you have had an uncomplicated labour previously. Otherwise, as for most able-bodied mothers, it is still quite difficult to arrange home births. If you are determined, seek advice from your local Supervisor of Midwifery.

Obstetric physiotherapist

An obstetric physiotherapist is a physiotherapist with specialist training in helping women to minimise aches and pains during pregnancy, labour and postnatally by teaching good posture and useful exercises. They work mainly in obstetric units of hospitals and often run antenatal classes early on in pregnancy to advise on adapting to your changing shape as pregnancy progresses. They can also advise on labour positions if your disability is such that you are concerned about the choices that will be available to you.

For a woman with a physical disability the obstetric physiotherapist can be a particularly useful support and may arrange to see you soon after your first antenatal appointment. If not, you could ring up the hospital and ask for an appointment with her yourself.

If your disability is such that you have a regular physiotherapist already, she may also be able to advise you on caring for your body through pregnancy.

Health visitor

You will probably meet your health visitor once during pregnancy and then again after your baby is born. The health visitor is part of the team of professionals (doctors, midwives, obstetric physiotherapists, etc.) which looks after the health of people in a particular doctor's practice or geographical area. She is a trained nurse with some midwifery experience and her job is to promote good health and prevent illness. For a new mother, she does this through regular developmental checks of the baby, advises on things like clothing, equipment, weaning and local childcare facilities. She is usually a mine of up-to-date information and can be a very useful source of support for a first-time mother.

Like any other professional, how useful any individual health visitor is to you, will depend on her personality, breadth of experience and how large her caseload is. It is an unfortunate fact that many health visitors spend more time trying to catch up on paperwork than visiting people who need their help. Try to help her to help you by telling her about how your disability affects your daily life and in which areas you feel you may need more support.

Health visitors may work from a GP practice, a health centre, or a clinic. A health visitor should come and visit you at home after the midwife stops coming and may continue to pop in on and off even if you cannot make it to her clinic. You can call her on the telephone for things that are worrying you, however trivial. She is well informed on DHSS benefits and may be able to arrange home-help in your early weeks at home if you need it. Because she is out and about a lot, you can usually only telephone her early in the morning (for example, between 9 and 10 am) and then again later in the afternoon. But you can always leave a message for her to contact you and she may even give you her home number in case of emergency. Don't be afraid to ask her for advice – that is her job and if it means a more content baby and more relaxed parents, then it is always worth it.

Occupational therapist

Occupational therapists work in hospitals and in the community to advise on adapting to ordinary life by showing ways of doing things that take your disability into account. She can advise on adapting the various rooms of your home and suggest any equipment that could make day to day chores easier. For example, for a wheelchair-user she could arrange for a ramp to be built, a special shower installed, electrical sockets raised – and all this may be paid for by local council grants.

You may have already been referred to an occupational therapist if your disability is such that you have needed one, but when preparing for a new baby it may be useful to renew contact with her. She may be able to offer useful advice on looking after a new baby and advise on what baby equipment to buy. If you do not already have contact with an occupational therapist, your GP can refer you.

Social worker

Social workers work for the local authority in which you live and can help parents with a disability in a variety of ways. You may be put in touch with a social worker attached to the hospital where you attend antenatal clinics, or you can contact the local authority department of social services yourself with particular queries.

The role of the social worker, which should be complementary to that of the other professionals involved in your care, is to provide practical and moral support should you need it, and, as with the other professionals, they will respect confidentiality.

Their practical support may be to do with housing, understanding social security benefits, local authority grants for special equipment, organising home-helps and so on. Their knowledge of the facilities available in your area and how to get access to them is what can make them of great use. They may also be able to help with family problems, for example, if you are facing opposition to your decision to have a child.

Mary Marlborough Lodge

This is a part of the Nuffield Orthopaedic Centre near Oxford and its work involves helping people with disabilities achieve independence as far as possible by suggesting new ways of doing things or appropriate equipment to enable a disabled person to carry out routine tasks with the minimum of effort and discomfort. It provides a residential service for mothers with disabilities to suggest practical tips for looking after a child.

The work of the Lodge is funded by the NHS and the women seen are referred by doctors, but anyone and everyone can initiate referrals – often it is social workers who do this. The Lodge likes to see women during the second or third trimester of pregnancy, and encourages partners to participate as much as they would like.

The current director outlined the following as the most common aspects of childcare that presented difficulties to women with a disability:

1. lack of balance
2. involuntary movements
3. anxiety
4. inexperience
5. lack of access from a wheelchair
6. lifting baby in and out of cot, on and off changing surface
7. safety of baby

A team of midwife, health visitor, therapists, social worker and doctor take part in the assessment and try to provide solutions tailored to the individual couple's situation and needs. Their long-standing experience and their access to a wealth of data regarding rehabilitation put them in a particularly strong position to do this.

Apart from Mary Marlborough Lodge, there are a number of other rehabilitation centres in hospitals around the country which can provide much of the same type of assessment and support.

Other assistance

Home-help

It may be possible to arrange a home-help for a few hours each week to do some shopping and cleaning from when you return home with the baby. Your health visitor or social worker can put you in touch with the local social services department to arrange this, or you can contact them directly. Look up the name of your council in the phone directory to find the social services' address or telephone number.

All women are entitled to home help for the first 10 days after they return home with a new baby, but in practice only those women who have expressed a need get one.

Care for an older child

If you have an older toddler already and find you have difficulty in coping, your health visitor or social worker may be able to get the child into a nursery during the day to give you some time off.

Social Security benefits

Disability related benefits

You will probably already be familiar with the benefits to which you are entitled, but it may be worth checking to see if there is anything extra at this stage. There is a variety of financial benefits available and a DHSS leaflet entitled *Help for Handicapped People* outlines them all. To get the leaflet, ask at your local library, post office or DHSS office or call Freephone DHSS. There is also a publication entitled *The Disability Rights Handbook* which outlines all entitlement.

Maternity benefits

Again, a number of leaflets are available from the same places as above, which outline DHSS benefits for mothers. See also *The Maternity Handbook* which outlines all state and employee benefits. All pregnant women are entitled to free dental treatment during pregnancy and for 1 year after the birth of the baby. Do take care of your teeth as hormone changes make gums and, therefore, teeth more vulnerable during pregnancy and breastfeeding.

All pregnant women are also entitled to free NHS prescriptions. You will need to complete a form (available from your GP) and send a Certificate of Confinement (proof that you are expecting a baby) from your GP or antenatal clinic along with it to the address on the form. You will be sent a certificate which you show every time you need dental treatment or a prescription. You may also be able to claim travel expenses to your antenatal appointments.

Once your child is born, you will be entitled to child benefit – currently £7–25 per child per week.

A final word on getting advice and information.

It is important to recognise that parents with a disability have a spectrum of needs just like any other parents. A few will need support most of the time, some will need help occasionally and others will manage perfectly well on their own.

As you will have seen, there is some overlap in the help that the various professionals can provide, so there is no reason why you should not get as comprehensive support as YOU may need – if you are prepared to ask for it. It may be helpful to identify one key professional (a health visitor or social worker, for example) who can coordinate the state support that is available to you.

Also, do remember to help professionals to help you more effectively by saying what you think your special needs are – these may not be the same as what an outsider perceives.

Try to build up a good two-way relationship with each professional you encounter, where you remain an expert on your own disability. You are then more likely to be able to keep your independence and dignity intact AND to get any support you may need.

Contacts

The Medical Advisory Service
10 Barley Mow Passage
London W4
Tel. 081-994 9874

This is a charitable organisation run by former nurses which will advise on all aspects of medical care. They do not give specific medical advice but help in explaining what your rights are as a patient and aim to help you communicate better with health professionals.

Association for Improvements in the Maternity Services (AIMS)
40 Kingswood Road
London NW6
Tel. 071-278-5628

This organisation can advise you of your rights as a consumer of the state maternity provisions. They can also be a support if you encounter any problems and need to formulate a complaint.

Local Citizens' Advice Bureaux can advise on all aspects of social security benefits.

Further reading

Evans, R. and Durward, L. (eds) (1984) *The Maternity Rights Handbook*, Penguin.

Robertson, S. (ed.) (1989) *The Disability Rights Handbook* (14th edn), Disability Alliance.

Available by post from:

Disability Alliance
25 Denmark Street
London WC2 8NJ
Tel. 071-240 0806

Chapter three

Your pregnancy

The first trimester (2 – 14 weeks)

So it's happening. You are pregnant and suddenly there is so much to plan and think about.

The coming months will probably bring many emotional ups and downs as you contemplate the arrival of The Baby. All pregnant women have moments when they worry whether the baby will be all right, whether they will cope, how he will affect their relationship with their partner, how he will affect their social life, their financial situation.

Having a child is an act of faith – on the whole you cannot predict what impact it will have on you and your life as this depends so much on the baby and on your own adaptability, stamina and confidence. All you can do is to look after yourself, get as well informed as possible, make the best practical preparations you can – and be realistically optimistic about the rest.

For a woman with a disability the major difference will be in the amount of planning you may need to do to prepare for each stage of pregnancy, your stay in hospital, and for looking after a new baby.

As far as the growing baby is concerned, a disabled woman is usually no different to an able-bodied woman. I have therefore not gone into any great detail about the normal physical process of pregnancy – there are a large number of good books on the subject.

Looking after yourself

There are a few general points about looking after yourself which apply to all pregnant women and which you will hear again and again:

Diet: eat regularly and try to eat a varied diet rich in protein and fresh fruit and vegetables. Avoid eating a lot of sweet or fatty things as these will cause you to put on too much weight – which you may not be able to lose later on and which may cause problems if your mobility is already restricted.

Smoking: if you have not already given up smoking do so now – for your own sake as well as for that of the growing baby.

Alcohol: an occasional glass of wine or a half of lager is probably harmless, but you should try to avoid drinking alcohol on a regular basis.

Drugs: don't take any drugs during pregnancy without first checking with your GP or specialist.

All these steps are to minimise the risk that you will miscarry, have a poorly nourished baby or one whose brain is damaged. They will also help to keep you feeling well.

Some common problems

Nausea: this is caused by the change in hormone levels in your body and most pregnant women experience nausea but to varying degrees. There are various things you can do to minimise the discomfort. One suggestion that seems popular is to eat some biscuits (water biscuits are particularly good) and have a cup of tea before you get out of bed. Another is to take vitamin B6 supplements, but check with your GP before consuming these in large quantities.

If it seems to you that you are bringing up everything you manage to eat, get reassurance from your GP. Even if you lose a little weight in the first few months you will make up for it later on, so there is usually no cause for alarm.

Tiredness: your body has embarked on a very strenuous course and is having to prepare itself to support two humans instead of just one, so it is hardly surprising that you tire so easily. There are steps you can take to minimise the tiredness:

1. Make sure you don't get anaemic. A blood-test is usually done at least once in this trimester and iron tablets and folic acid prescribed if you are found to be even slightly anaemic. Help yourself by eating a good mixed diet.

2. Learn to pace yourself and to build in short periods of relaxation throughout the day rather than collapsing into bed exhausted each night. Learning some simple techniques of relaxation now will help you

throughout your pregnancy and particularly in the early months after the baby is born.

3. Learn to say yes to help. If your partner has been reluctant in the past to help with housework and shopping, now is the time for change. What better time to get involved in the care of the unborn baby that is, after all, both of yours?

Many of the women I spoke to said that they regretted having been so fiercely independent and turning down help from friends and relatives when it was offered. There does seem to be a greater burden on women who are disabled to try to prove that they can cope all the time, for fear that people will question whether they are capable of looking after a child. Try to remind yourself that all pregnant women need to put their own well-being high on their list of priorities – a well mother is more likely to mean a well baby.

4. If you are going out to work, remember to avoid getting overtired. Find a few moments during the day to put your feet up or, if at all possible, have a breath of fresh air, which is often just as reviving. If your work involves sitting much of the day, be careful to maintain a good posture. If you can do so, get up and walk about every so often so as to maintain good circulation. If you cannot walk, take advice from a physiotherapist about ways of exercising your body.

Backache: this is a frequent problem for many pregnant women due to the many body changes taking place and the relaxing of the ligaments that accompanies pregnancy. If your disability is such that you are prone to backache anyway, you may well find that the problem is accentuated while you are pregnant (although there are some backaches which get better during pregnancy). There are a few precautions that all women should take:

1. Maintain as good a posture as you are able at all times. Use cushions to help support you when seated. When lifting things, the golden rule is to bend at the knees and hips, keep your back straight, lower yourself gently and hold the weight close to you as you raise yourself.

2. If your disability prevents you from doing this, the best thing is to avoid having to bend in the first place. Your home is probably already somewhat adapted to keep things at your height. Look again and see if there is anything that can be improved – now is the time to do it!

3. When sleeping, use pillows to support you – experiment until you find the most comfortable arrangement. If your disability permits it, remember to roll over on to your side to get out of bed.

Again, ask the obstetric physiotherapist for advice about these activities so that you can be shown the best ways of avoiding strain.

Bladder and bowel care: as the pregnancy proceeds, the growing baby will press on the bladder and also weaken pelvic floor muscles, so many women experience a need to empty their bladders more urgently and more frequently to avoid 'accidents'.

Pregnancy is also a time of increased risk from urinary tract infections, so you will need to keep up your fluid intake, be extra vigilant and get treatment immediately if you suspect that you have an infection.

If your disability is such that your bladder and/or bowel function is already affected, you may be concerned about the effects of pregnancy and childbirth. Again, every woman is different and needs to seek individual advice from her specialist. The general aim will be to minimise incontinence, prevent constipation, infections or distension of the bladder. The usual advice is to follow your normal routine unless there are medical reasons to do otherwise.

Urostomies, ileostomies and colostomies in pregnancy

You may have had surgery for one of the above as a result of your condition (for example, spina bifida, multiple sclerosis, cancer, a congenital abnormality) and may be interested to know what sort of problems may arise in pregnancy. The following information is adapted from a leaflet produced by the Urostomy Association.

Skin changes

Early hormonal changes of pregnancy can affect the skin and cause appliances not to stick so well, or to need more frequent changing. Skin wafers and extra skin adhesives can help remedy this problem.

Frequent changes of appliance or persistent leaks can lead to skin breakdown which needs to be avoided. There are preparations available which form a protective film over the skin and also help with adhesion of the appliance.

Stoma changes

As the abdomen enlarges, the urostomy, ileostomy or colostomy will also change shape, becoming more oval than circular. It is vital to maintain an accurate fitting of the appliance if damage to both skin and the stoma is not to occur.

33

Appliances with a precut hole will need to be changed for a different size; those where the hole is cut to fit will need to have a different pattern made to ensure an accurate fit. The stoma may become shorter or longer. If it shortens, it may retract below the flange of the appliance, causing more leaks, especially when you are lying down. It is worth trying an appliance with a softer, more mouldable flange if this becomes a serious problem.

Leaks occurring when you are lying down can also be due to the relative change in position of the stoma. As the abdomen enlarges, the stoma will tend to become more lateral. This will obviously make it more difficult to see the stoma when you are changing an appliance, so you will need to stand in front of a full-length mirror. It may also cause problems with lying down and sleeping, particularly later in pregnancy when it is difficult for most women to lie flat on their backs. Lying on the side of the stoma will make it leak; lying on the opposite side may cause problems in drainage of urine from the pouch into the night drainage system. Positioning yourself carefully with pillows seems to be the best solution.

Ultrasound scans

The gel that is spread on the abdomen for an ultrasound scan can cause problems to women with an ostomy by causing lack of adhesion. Take a spare appliance with you and after the scan, clean the area thoroughly with soap and water, before putting it on.

Scans in early pregnancy require a full bladder and therefore women with non-functioning bladders may not be able to have an effective scan. Ostomy bags can also cause difficulties for clear scanning. The person performing the scan will try to position you so as to work round any such difficulties, but it may take a bit of time.

Infection

If you have a urostomy you are more prone to infection in pregnancy and will need to be extra vigilant. Untreated urinary tract infection can lead to renal failure or premature labour so must be avoided.

Careful collection of an uncontaminated urine sample is important if infections are to be detected.To collect an uncontaminated sample, the appliance must be removed. The skin is then cleaned and either a clean catch sample of urine is collected from the stoma, or the stoma may be catheterised, using an aseptic technique. Urine spurts from the stoma at short intervals, so collection does not take very long.

Labour

In women with urostomies, obstruction of the ureter is not unusual in pregnancy. The growing uterus compresses the ureter (usually on the left) which crosses the vertebral column to reach the ileal conduit. This can cause the uterus to go into sympathetic contractions which may feel as though labour has started.

There should be few problems associated with an ostomy during actual labour. Appliances will obviously need to be changed after the birth because of the changed shape of the abdomen. After a Caesarean section, it is helpful for the theatre staff to change an appliance before a mother regains consciousness or full sensation. The abdomen will be quite sore for a couple of days after the operation, so it would be helpful not to have to prod it unnecessarily.

Postnatal period

Appliances will need to be changed frequently as the abdomen and the stoma regain their former shapes. Hormone changes may again affect the greasiness of the skin, causing adhesion problems.

It may be helpful to keep an empty bag ready before feeding, particularly breastfeeding, as an active baby can dislodge a full pouch or cause it to leak.

The second trimester (14 – 28 weeks)

This is usually the time in pregnancy that women enjoy most – the nausea has usually stopped, the 'bump' begins to appear and soon you begin to feel the baby moving around; your skin and hair begin to look better than ever and the tiredness and discomfort of the early weeks lessen. Now is the time to begin a gentle routine of breathing and exercise both to keep you fit and relaxed and to prepare you for childbirth itself.

Antenatal exercise

The three main aspects of exercise that obstetric physiotherapists concentrate on in pregnancy are as follows.

Pelvic floor muscles: these are the hammock of muscles around the vagina which are prone to slacken in pregnancy due to the additional weight of the baby. Simple exercises which focus on tightening and

35

relaxing these internal muscles can be done in any position and are vital to every woman as they help control stress incontinence (for example, leaking when coughing).

Abdominal muscles: these tummy muscles are being stretched as the baby grows and will remain flabby after giving birth unless you exercise during pregnancy and then again after the baby is born. There are a variety of exercises designed to strengthen the different muscles – for example, pulling your tummy in, slowly letting it go, and then repeating a few times throughout the day. These exercises can be done sitting or lying down. These are important muscles to strengthen as they help prevent backache.

Maintaining good circulation: exercises to maintain good circulation of the blood around the body are important in pregnancy because the changes caused by the growing baby can affect this. To avoid swelling of the legs and fingers, exercises that circle the arms, ankles and wrists will be suggested. If you are able to walk, then you will be advised to do so regularly. If the use of your legs is restricted, there are passive exercises with which you may already be familiar and which you should maintain during pregnancy.

All of these exercises can be modified for women with a particular disability and that is why you should seek advice. A physiotherapist can also advise on additional exercises that will help with your particular disability, for example, strengthening the muscles in the upper part of your body if you are in a wheelchair. The golden rule with all exercise is to tune into your body – do as much as feels comfortable, and stop if you feel any pain or become tired.

Many women with disabilities assume that, because they may not be able to do some of the exercises at antenatal exercise classes, there is no point in attending. Another common reason is that they feel embarrassed by the attention they get, or – worse – they are ignored because the teacher doesn't know how to deal with them. A further problem is that seating accommodation is usually scatter cushions on the floor rather than chairs, so women who have difficulty in getting down to the floor, or who are in wheelchairs, feel excluded. To aggravate the situation even further there is a national shortage of obstetric physiotherapists, so trained help is not always available.

If it is at all possible to attend classes (for example, if they are held in an accessible place either by a hospital, GP clinic, NCT group or yoga group) I would recommend doing so for the following reasons:

1. Even if you can only do some of the exercises, you will probably be able to adapt others to your own body's abilities, and do so under the watchful eye of someone experienced. You will learn breathing techniques to employ during labour and be given the opportunity to practise them.

2. You will learn relaxation techniques and there will be time to practise them at the end of the class – these are useful for pregnancy and labour (even if you are to have a Caesarean section), and for motherhood!

3. The class will provide a weekly outing to an activity designed just for you and your baby, and will help you think positively about the whole experience.

4. It will give you an opportunity to meet other women having babies around the same time as you and to make friends you may welcome after you have had your baby.

If you are unsure about how the teacher (usually a physiotherapist or midwife) will treat you, why not arrange to see her on your own first and discuss what your disability is and what you may or may not safely be able to do? Most teachers will welcome this approach by you, which gives them some time to think through how they can best help you – and, in future, others with your disability.

If you cannot manage the weekly classes it may still be worth having a chat with the teacher (and with your specialist if you have one) to see what exercises you can do at home.

Antenatal classes

You and your partner will probably be invited to attend weekly antenatal classes at the hospital from about 28 weeks, where you should be given advice on the following:

- The signs to expect when you go into labour
- Methods of pain relief
- Babycare and purchase of equipment
- What to bring into hospital

You will also be given an opportunity to visit the delivery suite and postnatal wards, and to ask questions about hospital policy so you know what to expect. Do try to attend these classes as you will pick up a lot of useful information and may feel encouraged to see how other parents are just as apprehensive and excited as you. You should hear about the classes by the 20th week of pregnancy; if you have not, contact the antenatal clinic or Directory of Midwifery Services at your local hospital.

Some mothers I spoke to chose not to attend antenatal classes because they assumed that they could get the information that is given there by reading books or asking their obstetrician or midwife. As for the shared experience, many women with disabilities felt they did not have that much in common with able-bodied women. An interesting example of this was the view of one mother with multiple sclerosis that such classes seemed to dwell on coping with the labour whereas she was more concerned with looking after the baby afterwards. As she was accustomed to pain she did not worry too much about coping with labour, and she regarded symptoms of a normal pregnancy (such as nausea) as a welcome sign that she was just like any other woman rather than as something about which to moan.

Other women assumed (often correctly) that antenatal classes would be held in inaccessible places or be more of an ordeal than they could cope with because of lack of suitable toilets, etc. If this is the case for you, do pass on your concerns to the antenatal teaching organiser – usually the Director of Midwifery Services at the hospital. They will almost certainly be able to tell you of alternative classes in a more accessible local health centre or midwives' clinic, or be able to organise a separate class for you and your partner on your own. Note also that the National Childbirth Trust runs local classes which prepare women and their partners for labour and parenthood. If you cannot get access to the classes, many NCT teachers will come to your home to give private tuition.

All these classes give you an opportunity to find out about the process of labour and the options available to you. For example, if you like the idea of a Leboyer-type birth (gently, in a quiet room with dimmed lights) you need to understand what to ask the midwives. Your disability should not automatically mean that you have no choices.

Postnatal support

If you have not already done so, find out about the facilities available in your area for mother-and-baby groups, etc. Contact the local social services department (number in the phone book), NCT group, etc. The local library or GP surgery often has information. It is also worth finding out from the social services department about Dial-A-Ride schemes, volunteer services such as Homestart – anything in your area that may help you, should you need it.

Preparation for the birth-day

At around 6 months prepare a list of things you will take to hospital and make sure you have bought anything that you don't already have. Leave the list somewhere where your partner can find it if you have to go into hospital earlier than expected. Otherwise, pack the case at around 2 months before the baby is due.

What to take: most hospitals provide a list, but remember that if you are to have a Caesarean, take more as you will be in longer. Also take some food as you may have the baby at a time when there are no meals available and you may be ravenous after the delivery. Take with you any drugs that you use routinely and give them to the midwife on admission to the hospital.

Discuss with your partner if you both want him to be at the birth. Most hospitals now accept the presence of the father and/or one other companion as normal practice. If he is to attend, talk about what he can do to help you – it may not be obvious to him. Discuss the methods of pain relief (see next chapter) and the ones you would prefer if there is a choice. Again, if you attend classes and antenatal check-ups together, he will be more in tune with how best he can support you.

If you are to have a Caesarean section under epidural your partner will be allowed to be present. If it is done under a general anaesthetic, he will not, but the baby will be given to him very shortly after, all being well.

Make sure you have worked out how you will get to the hospital. If you need to call an ambulance, remember to tell them that it is required for a woman in labour so they have the right equipment aboard – just in case! If you are in a wheelchair tell them this too.

The last trimester (28 – 40 weeks)

Around the 6th or 7th month start the preparations for your baby. Try to do these while you are still feeling well as you may be too tired if you leave it too late, or the baby may come earlier than you expect. Make sure you have a list of phone numbers of midwife, GP, hospital, etc. by your telephone in case of emergency.

Get help if you can and do the spring cleaning of the house, stocking up on household goods, preparing the baby's room, buying equipment, clothes and toiletries. Go gently – don't try to do too much in one go. Remember, if you're buying furniture or using mail order, that delivery may take several weeks, so allow plenty of time.

Get to know the health visitor (see Chapter 2) and ask for advice on what to get for the baby. Resist the temptation to buy lots of equipment before the baby is born. Think about your lifestyle and what suits you rather than what you are tempted by in the catalogues because it looks nice. If your partner is able-bodied and intends to help share in the care of the baby, you may have more flexibility in what suits you both. Ask your local occupational therapist to advise you about any adaptations to your home.

Preparation for the new baby

General: washing machine, food blender, any labour-saving devices you can afford and haven't already got – get them now if at all possible. Grants may be available in cases of financial hardship, and a social worker or health visitor may be able to advise you on these.

Somewhere to sleep: for the first few weeks, a small lined basket or carrycot. If you have mobility problems, an old pram that you can wheel from room to room may be useful even if you cannot comfortably use one out of doors.

Somewhere to change the nappies: you will probably change nearly 2000 nappies in the first year alone, so it is worth finding the most comfortable way for you to do so. Bear in mind the following:

- Is the height comfortable for you?
- Is the baby safe: can he roll off or pull anything dangerous on to himself?

Use a folded towel, or one of the wipeable mats you can buy, or you may find it easier to change the baby on your lap while wearing a plastic apron. A box or basket containing cotton-wool, wipes, cream, etc. can be kept beside you wherever you change the baby. You will need a pedal bin for disposable nappies, raised if necessary to make it easier for you to use, and also, later on, to keep it out of a crawling baby's reach.

If you live in a house with several floors, it may be worth considering having two nappy changing centres, one upstairs and one downstairs.

Somewhere to store clothes: shelves may be easier than drawers.

Clothes: avoid frilly things or fabrics that require handwashing and ironing. Ask friends and family to bear this in mind when buying presents. Envelope neck vests are easier to put on than the wrapover ones. Buy or get secondhand babygros – as many as possible (Mothercare, Boots, etc. do mail order) – it's amazing how many babies seem to get through each day in the early weeks! If fastening buttons is a problem, attach velcro fastenings to clothes. Velcro on towelling nappies is also a suggestion that may be of use. A warm shawl to wrap baby in may be more practical than fiddly cardigans.

Somewhere to bath the baby: don't invest in a plastic baby bath. The bathroom handbasin is usually a much more convenient place to bath the baby. If your partner is more able, this could be a task he might take on as his, bathing the baby in a basin or plastic bowl on the floor. You can buy sponge mats moulded to support a small baby in a basin of shallow water.

Or don't bath the baby – it's certainly not necessary to do this every day. It is perfectly possible to keep him clean with cotton wool and water and a gentle sponging while you hold him wrapped in a towel across your lap. This may be the best solution in the early days when you are still recovering and building your confidence in handling your baby. Later on a supervised splash is something that most babies enjoy.

Carrying the baby: a sling can be a very convenient way of carrying the baby, particularly in the early weeks before he gets too heavy. There are many on the market (not all of them good): look for one that has padding on the straps over the shoulders and is easy for you to get the baby in and out of. It is important to start using the sling as soon as possible after the baby is born so that he can get used to it. Most babies love being carried close to their parent's heart.

If choosing a pram or pushchair, consider the following:

- Weight
- Height of handles
- Ease with which it can be steered
- If it folds, can you make it do so while holding the baby?
- Comfort and safety: is it well sprung to cope with bumpy roads?
- Do the brakes work well?

Transporting the baby in a car: you should plan always to have the baby securely fastened in either a babyseat or (less satisfactory) a carrycot with straps. It is not safe to sit holding the baby – even a mildly abrupt halt can send him flying out of your arms, whether you're wearing a seatbelt or not. If you drive, a rear-facing baby seat, which is fastened by lap seatbelts and can be used in the front passenger seat, is less fiddly and strenuous than a carrycot in the back seat.

The last few weeks

You will probably be having more frequent antenatal checks either with your GP or at the hospital. Don't miss any – it is essential to monitor you and your baby carefully at this stage. It is during these last few weeks that the baby takes up his final position for delivery, ideally, head down in the pelvis. Sometimes he continues to lie bottom down or across your tummy. If he settles into the bottom down (breech) position, it could make a normal vaginal delivery difficult. In this case you may be examined with X-rays and ultrasound to see if your pelvis is big enough to try for a vaginal delivery, otherwise a date for a Caesarean section may be set.

Physical and practical problems due to your increased size may make it difficult for you to cope at home, in which case you may be admitted to hospital in advance of your due date. It should be remembered that, disability or not, the last few weeks are often uncomfortable. Disturbed sleep due to heartburn, the kicking baby and the impossibility of getting into a comfortable position, may leave you tired each morning. Other problems such as breathlessness, backache and piles can add to the discomfort.

Time may seem to go more slowly – people keep asking whether you've had the baby yet, and your own impatience grows. It is difficult to think of anything else. You may begin to feel ungainly, none of your clothes fit so you find yourself wearing the same things and feel as if you are bursting at every seam. Even if you and your partner have maintained any sort of sex life through your pregnancy, it becomes well-nigh impossible now! Apprehension, too, may return as the day of the baby's arrival suddenly becomes very real – will the delivery go all right, will the baby be all right . . . ? All these factors may contribute to both you and your partner becoming more tetchy and losing your temper over apparently trivial things.

Here are a few suggestions:

1. Stay active but remember to build in relaxation periods.

2. If heartburn is annoying you remember to eat little and often rather than having two or three big meals a day. Avoid eating rich or spicy foods if they seem to upset your stomach and try to eat your last meal at least 3 hours before you go to bed.

3. Keep in touch with friends/work colleagues – isolation at this stage is more likely to leave you feeling sorry for yourself.

Contacts

The following organisations can all provide advice about pregnancy and childbirth for women with an ostomy:

Urostomy Association
Buckland
Beaumont Park
Danbury
Essex
Tel. 024 541 4294

Ileostomy Association
Amblehurst House
Black Scotch Lane
Mansfield
Notts NG18 4PF
Tel. 0623 28099

Colostomy Welfare
38–39 Eccleston Sq
London SW1V 1PB
Tel. 071-828 5175

Further reading

There are many well-illustrated and comprehensive reference books about pregnancy now available. The *Marks and Spencer Book of Babycare* is particularly attractive and clearly presented. Another that has been recommended by many people is:

Chamberlain, G. (1987) *Pregnancy Questions Answered*, Churchill Livingstone.

Balaskas, J. (1983) *Active Birth*, Unwin Paperbacks.

If you are interested in natural childbirth despite any disability, this would make interesting reading.

Mitchell, L. (1987) *Simple Relaxation*, John Murray.

A highly recommended guide to different relaxation techniques.

Mary Marlborough Lodge (1989) *Disabled Mother* (6th edn), Mary Marlborough Lodge.

A guide to babycare products and equipment.
Available from:

Equipment for the Disabled
Mary Marlborough Lodge
Nuffield Orthopaedic Centre
Headington
Oxford OX3 7LD
Tel. 0865 64811

Another useful publication, *Aids and Adaptations for Parents with Physical or Sensory Disabilities*, is available by post (price US $15) from:

Dr T.A Conine
School of Rehabilitation Medicine
University of British Columbia
Vancouver BC
Canada V6T 1W5

Chapter four

In hospital

The vast majority of women in the UK have their babies in hospital where doctors are best prepared for any problems that may occur and where they have access to all the equipment and experienced staff that may be needed in an emergency. Few people like being in hospital and many of the mothers I spoke to found the problems of getting around, using the bathrooms, the noisy wards and staff that sometimes seem too busy to help, more difficult to handle than the birth.

Even if you have a completely straightforward birth, you are likely to stay in hospital for at least four days after a first baby and it may be many more if you have a Caesarean section or need to go into hospital in advance of your due date. So is there anything you can do to make your stay as comfortable as possible?

In the following guide I have incorporated some of the many suggestions that arose in my correspondence with mothers with disabilities – not all will be relevant but if you know about them you can decide what YOU would like to do.

Choosing a hospital

You may be given a choice of maternity hospitals (or hospitals with maternity wings) in your district health authority. Choose one that is easy to get to, but also find out whether any of the hospitals have obstetricians with expertise in your particular disability – it may be worth travelling a little further afield. Also, if you have the choice, you may prefer a smaller GP unit to a large, busy hospital. However, a smaller unit may not have as great a range of facilities. Find out the options, go and see the hospitals if possible, and then make a decision.

Getting to know the hospital

Your antenatal clinic appointments will make you familiar with getting to the hospital and, if you use a car, where best to park to minimise problems of access to the labour ward. If you attend the antenatal classes at the hospital, you will be given an opportunity to see the labour and postnatal wards. If you are not able to attend these classes, make a separate appointment to be shown around.

Visiting the labour and postnatal wards

Go with your partner and/or anyone else who will be with you during labour (for example, your mother or sister) – it will make it easier for them to help you on the day. Even if you know that you are to have a Caesarean section, becoming familiar with the layout of the maternity wards can make you more relaxed about the whole experience. As you go around, ask about any unfamiliar equipment, how the beds work (some are manually operated, others electrically to raise and lower them), and become familiar with the various uniforms of the staff – a bright smile and friendly interest will usually be met with helpful responses. You may even have the opportunity to get to know some of the midwives so that you are recognised when you come in to have the baby.

You can use this opportunity to ask about the range of pain relief offered by the hospital and to talk about positions for labour that you will be able to adopt.

If the postnatal ward looks as though it might pose difficulties, arrange to see Sister, who is a senior midwife in charge of the ward, and the physiotherapist. This will give you all the opportunity to discuss problems like access to toilets and bathrooms – perhaps it can be arranged for you to have a bed near them. If Sister does not seem to understand your disability, tell her briefly what you can and can't do and how you would like to be helped. It may be easier to do this now rather than to wait until after the birth, when you may feel weak and vulnerable. It will also give her the opportunity to prepare the rest of the staff for your stay and perhaps arrange for any extra equipment that they do not already have (such as a shower bench) that would make life easier for you.

You will also be allowed to bring in things to make you more comfortable, for example, a commode to use beside your bed, or special pillows to help you stay comfortable.

If you require a special diet, check whether the hospital can provide it adequately or whether you will need to supplement it from home. A hospital dietician should talk through your requirements and arrange for the kitchens to prepare appropriate food.

Many postnatal wards have a separate single room where you can be on your own. These are called amenity beds, and although the hospital may not be able to guarantee there will be one free on the day you come in, if you think you would like it, get this registered in your notes in advance. The advantages of an amenity bed are that it may be quieter and you may feel more comfortable out of the inquisitive gaze of the other mothers and their visitors. On the other hand, it may make you feel more isolated and miss out on the support that new mothers give each other and also the opportunity to see other mothers coping in the early days.

Find out what the hospital policy is on babies at night. Do babies stay by their mothers' beds or do they get taken away to a nursery to allow other mothers to get some sleep? If you intend to breastfeed you will need to check that you can stay close to the baby for night-time feeds. If you have mobility or sight problems, perhaps the night staff can bring the baby to you. This won't be an unusual request as many mothers who have had Caesarean sections or stitches have difficulty in getting around in the early days.

See whether the hospital cots are going to pose any problems – will you be able to lift the baby out on your own or will you have to depend on calling someone to do it for you? This is a problem that many disabled mothers have (and even able-bodied mothers who have had a Caesarean section). It may be possible for the hospital to get a cot with an adjustable base so that it can be lowered to the level of your own bed.

Check the visiting hours and how flexible they are. For example, many postnatal wards have extended visiting hours for the fathers but no one else. This gives you more time together and a chance for the father to get to know the baby and learn to handle him too. See whether arrangements can be made to permit your partner or relative to spend more time helping you outside the normal visiting hours, if this would make things more manageable.

Birthplans

A number of mothers I have spoken to suggested writing a short birthplan outlining your own disability, special needs, and your choices regarding how your labour is managed. They found it reassuring to know that their wishes were clearly laid out in writing so that they would not have to become involved in lengthy discussions while in the throes of labour. To be of maximum use, the birthplan should be discussed with midwives and doctors at your antenatal check-ups so that your options are clear BEFORE you go into labour. Give a copy of the birthplan to the doctor so that it is included in your notes and can be referred to when you are admitted to hospital to have your baby.

Admission day

You may be advised to come into hospital in advance of your due date if there are any special reasons why you need to be closely monitored. Otherwise you will come in on the day you go into labour or on the day that has been agreed for an induction or Caesarean section. Your partner, or anyone else you have chosen to attend the birth, can help by representing your wishes to the hospital staff while you are coping with the pain, using your breathing techniques and so on.

Admission following onset of labour

During your antenatal classes you will have discussed the signs that indicate that labour has begun. The most obvious of these is regular painful contractions across your abdomen. For a first baby, the labour will last several hours, so there is usually no hurry about getting to hospital – unless you have been advised otherwise.

Once you arrive at the labour ward you will probably be met by a midwife who will ask you about your contractions, whether your waters have broken, etc. She will then take your blood pressure and examine the state of your cervix to see how far dilated you are. You need to be 10 cm dilated before you are ready to push, and the first 5 cm take a lot longer than the second. She will also check the baby's heartbeat and attach to your tummy a device for monitoring contractions, called a cardiotacograph. This may be removed after 20 minutes or so, or kept on throughout labour.

If you have bladder incontinence due to your disability, an indwelling catheter will be placed early on in labour to maintain continuous drainage. It will probably be kept there for a few days after the baby is born. This is something that will have been discussed antenatally, and your obstetrician may arrange for you to see a urologist after the birth.

Pain relief

At this point the midwife will discuss methods of pain relief. Again, you will be told about these during antenatal classes and may already have some idea of your preferences. Don't be too rigid about this, though – it is difficult to know how you will cope with labour pain until it starts.

There are many non-medical forms of pain relief which you may have heard about. These include relaxation and breathing exercises as taught at antenatal classes. Such techniques can be very helpful but you do need to have practised them before the labour day. Acupuncture and TeNS (Transcutaneous Nerve Stimulation) are other less common forms of pain relief which you might want to investigate. Massage by your partner or midwife can be very relaxing too. If you can comfortably sit in a warm water bath, this may be a helpful way of coping with the pains in early labour.

The most common forms of medical pain relief offered by the hospital are:

Pethidine: this is a pain-killer given by injection which takes about 20 minutes to start working. It is designed to reduce the pain of contractions while leaving the mother awake. One often-quoted side-effect is that it may make the newborn baby very sleepy, but this only happens if the pethidine is given within an hour or so of the baby being born. A more common problem is that women are affected differently by pethidine – some find it doesn't make any difference to the pain at all.

Epidural anaesthetic: this is an anaesthetic given by inserting a fine plastic tube in the epidural space around the spinal cord. An epidural can completely remove sensation from the lower part of the body, but it needs to be started before labour is too far advanced and needs to be topped up throughout until a little while before you are ready to push – the sensation is then allowed to return. This is usually a very effective form of pain relief but has the disadvantage that you are likely to be more restricted in your movements as the tube has to remain inserted. There is also a greater likelihood that you may require a forceps delivery.

Entonox (often called gas-and-oxygen): this is a mixture of nitrous oxide and oxygen, kept in a cylinder and inhaled through a mask placed over the nose and mouth. The mixture takes a few seconds to work, so you need to inhale as soon as a contraction starts in order to obtain maximum relief when it peaks. A few women find it does not help, or they do not like the smell, but for others it is a very immediate, controllable and safe form of relief.

It may be that your particular disability means that you should avoid certain forms of pain relief – for example, you may not be able to have epidural anaesthetic if you have a neurological condition (such as epilepsy or multiple sclerosis) or spine damage. Again, find this out in advance.

Women experience labour pains very differently, but the most painful time is usually at the end of the first stage (before you are ready to push). One woman described this: 'I didn't know it was possible to be in such pain and still live!'; another: 'I kept waiting for it to get worse but it was all over before it became unbearable.' There is no doubt that your own attitude and ability to remain unfrightened and relaxed will help minimise the pain. Try to remember to use your breathing exercises to relax and distract you and to think of the pain as something creative that is bringing you closer to meeting your child.

Making links with the labour ward staff

Details of your disability should be recorded in your notes so that all staff dealing with you during labour should know about it. If your midwife seems ignorant of how your disability affects you, your partner should calmly explain it. Avoid any confrontations – you have enough on your plate!

The midwife is a highly trained professional and is there to help you deliver the baby safely. She will stay with you until the baby is born (unless your labour goes on across a shift-change) and you should have plenty of time to build a good relationship. If the disability is particularly severe a doctor rather than the midwife may perform the delivery.

In my correspondence, midwives were almost unanimously praised. It may be that your midwife has not come across anyone with your disability before, so if there are any special precautions that she seems unaware of, your partner should point them out. These may include taking extra care in positioning you, avoiding the use of stirrups and so on.

One common problem that women with a variety of disabilities have mentioned to me was how labour staff sometimes ignored them – addressing questions to the partner or to each other. This is the old 'Does he take sugar?' problem; it can be very hurtful and undermines confidence. Again, your partner or other companion in labour should calmly point out that all communication should be addressed to you. In the delivery room there may be several people coming in and out other than the midwife. At least one doctor will see you, maybe the consultant or senior registrar (the two most senior doctors), and you may also be asked whether you mind a student observing. You can refuse – but remember that students have to learn somehow. My own feeling is that if the student doctor (or midwife) is prepared to spend a little time getting to know you during labour rather than just coming in for the actual birth, I would not object. However, this is a very personal matter and perhaps you should discuss it with your partner beforehand so that it doesn't get in the way on the day. Everyone should identify themselves to you and your partner – if you are in any doubt as to who someone is, ask!

Labour positions

If you are able to move around at all, you may find trying different positions helps with the pain during contractions, for example, leaning against your partner, midwife or a chair, swaying or circling your hips. The most common position for women in labour is sitting upright (not lying) on the bed. If there is a particular position that you need to avoid (for example, lying on a weak leg), tell the midwife at the beginning. Using foam wedges, she can help you adopt a variety of positions until you find the most comfortable one.

If your disability involves immobility, paralysis, weakness, impairment of sensation, poor circulation or poor nutrition, there is an increased risk of pressure sores, so more care will be required in positioning during labour and then on the postnatal ward. Incontinence can also contribute to skin breakdown, since moisture causes skin maceration and faster bacterial growth. Pressure sores can develop within 3 hours but may take months to heal, so it is important that they are prevented.

You will probably already be familiar with preventive care at home, and the midwives caring for you should also be aware of special care required. Bony prominences such as elbows, coccyx, shins, etc. may need extra padding, especially when the delivery table, stirrups, and straps are used.

Repositioning to relieve pressure should be scheduled every 30 – 60 minutes during labour, and extra pillows may be used to allow you to do so independently.

Deliverance!

At intervals throughout your labour, the midwife (and/or doctor) will be checking your blood pressure, the baby's heartbeat, your contractions and how far your cervix has dilated. When it is fully dilated your contractions will seem to be coming almost continuously and your midwife will tell you when you are ready to push. You can best help your body push the baby out if you can use the breathing techniques (as taught in the antenatal classes) with the guidance of the midwife and your partner.

As the baby's head makes its way out, your perineum (the whole area around your vagina) will stretch. Sometimes, particularly for first babies, it doesn't stretch enough and may tear. The midwife may notice this and do an episiotomy (a surgical cut) before the tear occurs. Episiotomies are not done as routinely as they have been in the past, as the evidence that they heal better than tears has been largely discounted.

An episiotomy is also done if forceps are required because your baby has not progressed down the birth canal and has become distressed in any way. Forceps look very large and daunting but, in fact, are very safe, and only a small part of the instrument is actually inserted.

Finally, your baby arrives. The midwife quickly notes his appearance and whether he is breathing or hindered by the cord.

You should mention to your midwife that when the baby arrives, unless he is distressed or needs help, you would like him to be given to you straight away, if that is what you want.

If you intend to breastfeed, you may like to let the baby suckle straightaway – it'll probably be comforting for both of you after all the exertion and there is some suggestion that this helps you deliver the placenta more easily. Many women do not remember delivering the placenta – it usually happens with another few contractions while you are still absorbed by the baby. Just occasionally it gets stuck and the midwife has to take action to remove it.

If you need stitches a doctor (sometimes the midwife) will do them – again, they should be vigilant about positioning if you have spinal problems, as stitching usually involves having your legs up in stirrups; however, it may be done while lying on your side. Your partner may be able to hold the baby while this is happening.

If everything has gone smoothly, you and your partner will be left alone for about an hour just to be with the baby and each other.

You will then be helped into a wheelchair or trolley and a porter may accompany you to the postnatal ward. You will probably be exhausted, thirsty, hungry, and dazed by the feat you have just accomplished. Many mothers are exhilarated and just want to look at their baby. If it has been a particularly difficult labour, you may feel numb and tired: don't worry – there will be plenty of time to get to know the baby and, in the meantime, you can both sleep.

Your partner will be able to stay with you for a little while, even if it is night-time. He can ensure that all your belongings are put away in your bedside cabinet and any essential equipment such as crutches or transfer boards are easily accessible. He can also check that the staff know of your disability and any special requirements that you have. And then he can go home and get some well-deserved rest too.

Caesarean sections

You may be told at some stage during your pregnancy that it would be safest for both you and the baby to have a Caesarean delivery. There may be a number of reasons for this: if your spine or pelvis is misshapen in any way or your pelvis is too small to allow the passage of the baby's head; or if you have heart problems and may not be able to stand the exertion of labour. You may not discover you are to have a Caesarean until much later, possibly because the baby is lying across or breech instead of head down. Or it may be an emergency because the baby gets into an awkward position or becomes distressed during labour and has to be taken out quickly. A surgeon can remove the baby in a matter of minutes.

Whatever the reason for the Caesarean section, remember you will be no less a perfect mother, and the well-being of both you and the baby is the most important consideration. You may miss out on labour pains but you will have your share of pain and discomfort after the baby is born!

Caesarean sections are usually carried out under general anaesthetic which means you don't feel anything and are not at all aware of what is going on until you come round, shortly after the baby is born. You may feel groggy for anything up to 2 days depending on how quickly your individual metabolic system clears the anaesthetic out.

A large minority of Caesareans are now carried out under epidural anaesthesia. A needle is inserted at the base of your spine while you lie on your side, a fine tube is attached and the anaesthetic injected. The dose is maintained by top-ups for as long as necessary. You remain fully conscious and feel no pain, but you do feel the tugging sensations as the surgeon goes to work. The advantages are obvious: you can meet your baby straight away, your husband can be present, and you won't feel as groggy afterwards as under a general anaesthetic.

The epidural technique requires longer to work and sometimes the relief it gives is incomplete. Also, epidural anaesthesia may not always be given if you have multiple sclerosis or other neurological illness/spinal damage. Babies born under either form of anaesthesia are equally healthy if the procedures are carried out correctly.

However your baby is delivered, the surgeon will remove the afterbirth, tidy up and sew you up again – all this can take up to an hour. For the next couple of days you will be monitored carefully. If you need it, you may have a catheter placed to drain your bladder until your own sensations return.

Abdominal gas pains are often a problem – ask the obstetric physiotherapist for advice on how to relieve these.

Special care baby units

In some instances a baby will have to be monitored closely after birth. This could just be a precaution or more obviously necessary (for example, if the baby is born prematurely and needs to be supported artificially until his lungs are mature enough to function on their own). In either case, he will be kept in the Special Care (or Neonatal) Unit where specially trained nurses will take care of his every physical need and keep a close watch on him. These nurses are usually midwives so they will be just as understanding of your needs as the mother.

When you see the baby, he may look small and fragile, and the equipment may look daunting. Ask to have it explained to you and also ask if you may hold him, which may help to make him seem more like yours again! If you want to breastfeed, ask to be shown how to express your milk until he is ready to take it direct.

On the postnatal ward

Whether you have had a vaginal or a Caesarean delivery, the first few days afterwards may seem very strange as you may be tired and uncomfortable and at the same time trying to come to terms with the care of a new human being.

If you have had a Caesarean section you may be in a lot of pain, although pain-killers can ease the discomfort to some extent. You may find handling the baby well-nigh impossible and, if you are breast-feeding, you may need help to latch the baby on and then to take him off again. All things are possible but may seem nightmarishly difficult for the first few days.

Take everything gently and slowly. Tell the midwives if the discomfort suddenly gets worse, and ask for advice about urinating or opening your bowels, if stitches or catheters seem a problem. Having a baby certainly puts you back in touch with basic bodily functions! Remember that all new mothers, disabled or not, experience some discomfort, and that it does pass.

If your disability allowed you to walk befor the baby was born, you will be encouraged to start moving around a few hours after the birth. Learn how to raise and lower the bed and ask for advice about the best way to get in and out of bed, if this has become a problem. A physiotherapist usually comes round the ward soon after the birth to suggest gentle exercises you can do to help speed up recovery – ask her for any special suggestions that take your disability into account.

Losing a baby

Unfortunately not all pregnancies have happy endings and the death of a baby at any stage is a tragedy that a few parents have to face. It is very rare and the cause can often – but not always – be discovered. Feelings of guilt often accompany such a sad event, but it is very rarely anyone's fault, least of all the mother's.

Most hospitals offer photographs of the stillborn baby to the parents and help to organise a proper funeral so that parents and relatives can mourn the loss of the child fully. It is important to acknowledge the death in this way, as you have lost a real person.

You may be asked permission to allow a post-mortem examination of the baby to help ascertain what was wrong. It is entirely up to you whether you agree to this, but bear in mind that the results may be helpful if you embark on another pregnancy.

Learning babycare

During your stay on the postnatal ward you will be shown how to change your baby's nappy, how to keep him clean by topping-and-tailing (wiping face and bottom with dampened cotton wool) and bathing, and you will be given help in feeding him, whether by breast or bottle. Many of the mothers I spoke to described feelings of awkwardness and acute self-consciousness during these sessions and said they only relaxed when they got home and were able to sort out their own ways of doing things away from the ward staff and other mothers.

A hospital occupational therapist may be able to help with suggestions that take into account your disability. Midwives and nursery nurses are usually keen to help – they have chosen their jobs because they like babies and like helping new mothers – so take advantage of their expertise. There are usually several periods during the day when they can be called upon for advice. If the group sessions are awkward for you, ask the Sister if she can arrange for you to have one on your own. This may give you the opportunity to try out your own adapted ways of caring for the baby and give the midwife an opportunity to offer helpful suggestions too. What you need is to build confidence and to get information about products and safety.

Bottle or breast?

If at all possible you should try to breastfeed as this is the best form of nourishment for the baby. However, there are times when bottle-feeding may seem preferable and you may get conflicting advice about which would be best for you. See Table 4.1.

Very few disabilities actually make breastfeeding impossible. The only deterrent might be drugs you are taking getting into the breast milk. If this is a worry, check with the doctor (see box). You may need a bit of help in getting the breastfeeding established, but if you want to breastfeed, do persist.

Risks from drugs in breast milk

Most drugs taken by the mother are excreted in breast milk but are usually present in tiny amounts that are unlikely to harm the child. Where practicable all drugs should be avoided during breast-feeding but if they are necessary you should seek advice from your doctor who can check the up-to-date information on their safety before advising you.

Table 4.1

Breast		
Advantages		*Disadvantages*
No bottles to carry around, sterilise and heat.		No one else can help with feeding the baby unless you are able to express milk – which is not always easy.
Is readily available.		
Mother's milk helps baby's immunity.		
May help avoid certain allergies.		May be inadvisable if you are taking certain drugs.
May help you lose weight.		May be uncomfortable due to your disability.

Bottle		
Advantages		*Disadvantages*
You know how much the baby is drinking.		You need to be stringent about bottle hygiene and making up formula correctly.
Partner or other help can feed baby. Enables father to be close to baby too.		
May be more comfortable for you.		

Always sit, or lie, comfortably, using pillows if necessary to support the baby and prevent you from stooping to feed him. Cracked nipples are due to bad positioning – do make sure the baby is latched on properly and ask for help with this. Although it is natural to breastfeed, it is not always straightforward in the early days and you may feel overwhelmed by the conflicting advice you receive.

Early problems, such as sore nipples, soon disappear if correctly dealt with, and most women enjoy breastfeeding. Don't be afraid to ask for help, even when you are back home. The health visitor should be able to help you with breastfeeding problems or you can contact one of the National Childbirth Trust breastfeeding counsellors (you don't need to be a member of the NCT to ask for this advice). Remember that the more the baby sucks, the more milk you will produce, so, if you think the baby is not getting enough, let him suck as much as he wants to get your supply up.

There are many myths about breastfeeding, most of which are false. These include stories of women not being able to breastfeed because they don't have enough milk or their breasts are too small. The misinformation is further aggravated by the fact that the generation of mothers of women now producing children were told that bottle was better than breast and so they cannot show their daughters how to breastfeed. If your mother was a product of this generation (1950s), be warned.

However, having extolled the virtues of breastfeeding, there are likely to be instances where you may decide bottle-feeding is better for you all, and as long as you hold the baby close he will be quite content to get his food from a bottle. Ask for advice about which formulas to try – if there is a history of allergies in your family, you may be advised that cow's milk-based formulas should be avoided and soya milk ones used instead. Health visitors also now advise that babies should not be given ordinary cow's milk until they are over a year old as it is not as rich in vitamins and minerals as either breast milk or formula and can cause allergies.

Further reading

NMAA (1982) 'Where there's a will, there's usually a way', *A Guide to Breast-feeding where the Mother has a Disability*, NMAA. Available from:

NMAA (Nursing Mothers Association of Australia)
PO Box 231
Nunawading
Victoria 3131
Australia.

Consumers Association (January 1983) 'Drugs which can be given to nursing mothers', *Drugs and Therapeutics Bulletin*, Consumers Association.

Messenger, M. (1986) *The Breastfeeding Book*, Century.

Kitzinger, S. (1989) *Breastfeeding your Baby*, Dorling Kindersley.

A selection of leaflets on all aspects of breastfeeding is available from:

The National Childbirth Trust
Alexandra House
Oldham Terrace
London W3 6NH
Tel. 081-992 8637.

Chapter five

You and your child

Coming home from hospital

Coming home with a fragile-looking newborn baby may seem terrifying, or you may just be relieved to get home to familiar surroundings. A practical point: do remember to have the baby securely fastened in a carry cot or baby seat if you are coming home in a car.

In terms of medical care the transfer from hospital to home after having a baby is the best organised of any – the hospital automatically notifies the health visitor and community midwife and the latter should call at least once in the first 24 hours that you are home. If you don't get a visit, call the hospital and ask them to check.

For the first few days a community midwife will come to your home to check your blood pressure, any stitches, and your general health, and also to weigh and examine the baby. The baby's umbilical cord will drop off in these early days and she will keep the area clean to avoid infection.

Don't assume that because you're home you can live life at the pace you did before you were pregnant. You are still vulnerable to tiredness and infection, particularly if you have had stitches. If you have had a Caesarean section, it may be a few months before you will feel normal again. If you have had a vaginal delivery it will probably be at least 6 weeks before your body seems vaguely familiar again. Remember, too, that tiredness is an ever-present feature of bringing up children, and you cannot hope to do too much at first. So, take it easy. The ideal is just to enjoy getting to know your baby and forget about housework and everything else. Eat simple foods, such as nourishing soups, that don't involve too much effort. Remember you need to look after yourself as well as the baby. If you are breastfeeding, you won't produce as much milk if you let yourself get exhausted.

Deter visitors, particularly large numbers at a time that have to be catered for. There will be plenty of time for them to meet the baby later. A helpful mother or mother-in-law may be a wonderful lifesaver, but make sure you agree who's in charge! Different approaches to child rearing (for example, leaving the baby to cry or picking him up straight away) can give rise to a lot of ill-feeling if not discussed properly.

Encourage helpers to fit in with your ways of caring for the baby, particularly in your own home. Any help with housework and cooking and shopping should be accepted in the early weeks so that you can devote yourself to the baby and to recovering your own health. Your partner needs time to get to know the baby too, so make sure he's not missing out.

Finally, the much talked about 'baby blues'. It is estimated that up to 60 per cent of mothers experience depression in the early days after the birth of the baby, and the most likely cause is your hormone balance going through all sorts of readjustments. Do not blame your disability and try not to expect too much of yourself at this stage. For the majority of women the low should pass fairly soon – if you feel it going on for weeks, seek advice from your GP.

Feedback

At some point in the first few weeks try to find some time to sit down and write a letter to the obstetrician or ward Sister saying 'thank you' if you have been well-treated, and offering suggestions if you feel there is anything that could have been done better. This feedback is important and enables other mothers in the future to have better treatment too. If you have any cause for serious complaint, seek advice from AIMS about the most effective procedure.

As the baby grows older . . .

Looking after a child can be a very lonely business and this can become even more of a problem if you have trouble getting out and going to mother-and-baby groups, baby clinics, and so on. A good health visitor is likely to keep in close touch with you if this is the case. If you can find a group that you can get to, it's well worth the effort. Otherwise, how about inviting friends made antenatally over to your place one afternoon a week? It will help you avoid becoming isolated and your baby will soon begin to take an interest in other babies too.

Childcare

There is no doubt that help with childcare is one of the main challenges facing any mother, but for a woman with a disability it is what can make the difference between enjoying the experience of bringing up a child or going through hell. There are two main problems about getting help: one is the lack of availability and the second is the cost. State provision of nurseries is still patchy and over-subscribed but, depending on the extent of your disability and social circumstances, you may get priority over other mothers. Your health visitor or social services department should be able to advise you on the provisions in your area.

Other options to explore are schemes such as Community Service Volunteers or Homestart whose volunteers can help housebound parents in practical ways such as providing outings for children. One suggestion I also received was to ask at local colleges of further education about nanny trainees who, as part of their course work, are required to spend a day or two a week looking after a child at home. Ask at your local Citizens' Advice Bureau for details of volunteer organisations that operate in your area.

Childminders, private nurseries, and nannies are the other options, depending on the money you have available to you. Ask your social services department about any financial assistance to which you may be entitled. The Independent Living Foundation also offers grants to cover childcare costs for those parents with disabilities who are eligible for attendance allowance.

Practical tips on childcare and equipment

Just as with other aspects of daily life, bringing up a child when you are disabled requires continual trial-and-error experimentation with adaptations to see what works for YOU. It is very difficult to plan ahead – you cannot know how you will catch a crawling baby until your baby starts to crawl, or how you will lift a 2-stone toddler when you are in a wheelchair or have weakness in your arms.

In the individual chapters on specific disabilities in Part 2 I have included tips that have been passed on by other disabled mothers. At the time of writing this book, a massive compendium of such tips is being compiled by Kate Liffen, a mother with multiple sclerosis who belongs to the NCT Disability Working Group. No publication date has yet been set but she has expressed a willingness to share what information she has gathered with anyone who wishes to contact her in the meantime, through the NCT Contact Register.

I recently came across the work of a Californian group called Through the Looking Glass which has been set up to promote understanding and support for parents with disabilities. For one of their research projects, video recordings have been made over two or three years to show how very small babies adapt to their parents' disabilities. There were a lot of very encouraging findings which show how even tiny babies can learn to cooperate with tasks such as lifting, or lying still while having their nappy changed by a disabled parent. Another observation was that disabled parents spent more time playing, talking, and generally communicating with their young babies as a result of these tasks requiring more time and cooperation with the baby – a positive benefit. As the babies grew older they quite happily accepted their parents' disability as a normal part of their lives. Mothers with mobility or balancing problems developed all sorts of cooperation games with their crawlers and toddlers.

I think a lot more work of this kind needs to be done in the UK and made widely available on video so as to provide more positive images of disabled parenting to both prospective parents and health professionals. Many of the mothers I have spoken to have described their frustrations and anxieties about managing the practical aspects of looking after a baby or toddler, only to realise later that this is a very short-lived stage in being a parent. Many wished they had managed to keep a perspective on it at the time rather than feeling guilty and inadequate. While safety and physical well-being are obviously important in looking after a child, it is easy to forget the importance of developing a stable and loving relationship with him.

Further reading

Hale, G. (1979) 'The Disabled Parent', *The Source Book for the Disabled*, New York: Paddington Press.

This illustrated chapter offers a practical guide to babycare, with sections on equipment, lifting and carrying, safety and cooperative behaviour.

Kehm, V.C. (n.d.) *Childcare for Physically Limited Mothers*, pamphlet no. EC 71–2209, University of Nebraska: Home Management Rehabilitation.

An illustrated guide with practical advice, hints, and techniques for the disabled mother.

Lunt, S. (1982) *A Handbook for the Disabled. Ideas and Inventions for Easier Living*, New York: Charles Scribner's Sons.

Moore, J. (1981) 'Can a wheelchair-bound woman have a baby?', *Accent on Living* 25:79–81.
Written by a mother with polio, this includes a list of 'Ten tips on Disciplining Children from a Wheelchair'.

General childcare

Jolly, H. (1988) *The Book of Childcare*, Unwin Paperbacks.

Leach, P. (1989) *Baby and Child*, Penguin.
The above are just two of the many general books on childcare that many parents have found useful over the years, but there is no reference to disability in either.

Parent and *Mother and Baby* magazines (the latter is available on cassette) are useful reading in the early months with a new baby. Reading about other mothers' problems is often helpful and the magazines are a useful source of tips and news on new products, especially if you cannot get out to the shops much. Also, a quarterly newsletter, 'Newsletter for Parents with a Disability', is produced by the National Childbirth Trust and is available from the London headquarters as listed previously.

Through the Looking Glass (American Organization for Disabled Parents) produces a regular newsletter available from 801 Peralta Ave, Berkeley, California 94707, USA.

Chapter six

Support from health professionals

Attitudes towards people with disabilities have slowly improved over the last twenty years and, on the whole, health professionals are much more positive about supporting those disabled women who want to have children. From my correspondence it seems clear, however, that problems do still arise, and I thought it worthwhile to include this chapter to help prospective mothers prepare for what they might face and also to give health professionals an insight into where they might improve the service they provide.

My own research has suggested that the onus is still very much on the mother to ASK for information and any special provisions she may require, rather than expecting to be given it automatically. This is not necessarily a bad thing as long as you, the mother, know that this is the case – every woman with a disability is unique in her degree of handicap, her desire for information and also the number of special provisions she may need.

The rest of this chapter is addressed to health professionals, but I hope that prospective parents reading it will be better equipped to demand the best care possible from the professionals around them.

Understanding disability

To an outsider the obvious problems that a woman with a mobility or sensory disability faces are her practical difficulties in getting in and out of buildings, problems of transport, and, sometimes, economic difficulties. What is often not considered is that the most damaging barriers are the negative attitudes of other people, particularly amongst health professionals. Many people who are otherwise considerate demonstrate a surprising degree of ignorance and insensitivity when dealing with a person with a disability. This often leads to direct or indirect discouragement from the option of parenthood and, if such a woman becomes pregnant, may lead to an undermining of her confidence and even poor care.

Some causes of negative attitudes

Distaste at the idea of the sexuality of the disabled

This is a common but often unvoiced prejudice. Part of the problem arises because some people find it difficult to imagine finding a person with an externally visible disability sexually attractive; this in turn, I think, is due to unfamiliarity and the lack of disabled people in the media and advertising, in other words, in the places from which most people derive their images of attractiveness. Getting to know someone in their home environment and seeing them with their friends and loved ones may help to see the person beyond the disability. The association for the Sexual and Marital Problems of the Disabled (SPOD) can organise seminars for professional groups to help overcome ignorance and prejudice.

Feeling uncomfortable in the presence of a disabled person

Should you open the door, should you offer to push someone in a wheelchair, should you offer someone with shaky movements a cup of coffee? This awkwardness is often due to ignorance of the capability (rather than the disability) of the individual, and can usually be overcome by asking, in a straightforward manner, what the particular person would prefer.

Misconceptions

- Disabled people don't have normal intelligence
- All disabled women have to have Caesareans
- Disabled people are dependent
- A disabled person is an ill person
- The child is at risk
- A disabled person cannot be a proper parent

The above statements are all false in the majority of instances but they are common misconceptions arising from a failure to see the person with a disability as an individual. The only way to overcome this is to take the trouble to get to know the individual person and how their disability affects them. Rather than looking only at what they can't do, try to get to know what they can do and how. Prejudice means 'pre-judging' – try to avoid this!

What can the health professional do?

To a health professional, the environment of a hospital or clinic is a familiar and unthreatening one. To a disabled woman and her partner, such environments are often unsettling: they are places where she cannot be sure of her autonomy and they may be associated with unpleasant memories due to previous medical treatment.

When such a woman and her partner meet a health professional (who usually has all the trappings of authority such as a uniform and a technical language), she is just another case on his list. But for her, this pregnancy is one of the most significant events ever to take place, and the birth of her child will have repercussions on every aspect of her life thereafter.

The couple may be intimidated by the fear of being judged as unfit to be parents and so may be reluctant to ask for advice from the health professional. Before she has even opened her mouth to speak, the disabled woman is already at a disadvantage in this relationship – the technology, the language, the environment are all alien, but the body and the life are hers.

As a starting point, it is important for health professionals to recognise this inherent imbalance in power and to try to redress it. How the woman's pregnancy, birth and postnatal period are managed by health professionals will affect the confidence and success with which she embraces the challenges of motherhood. It is therefore crucial to pay heed to the psychological needs of the woman and her partner, as well as the practical ones, and to see yourselves as enablers rather than carers.

A positive approach to motherhood for the disabled woman

The ideal that should be aimed for is: 'How can we work together as a team to facilitate a healthy, educated pregnancy, a positive birth experience, and a confident mother?'

1. Team approach: there should be good communication between professionals caring for the woman.

2. The health professional can encourage the disabled woman to be a responsible parent by providing her with information and by involving her in decisions to do with all aspects of parenting.

3. Since working with a disabled woman is not an everyday occurrence for obstetricians, midwives, antenatal teachers, and hospital staff questions will arise that require some research. I hope some answers will be found in this book, and others by contacting rehabilitation centres, teaching hospitals, and disability organisations.

4. The woman and her partner will welcome frankness on the part of the doctors and midwives when asked for information about her disability and self-care. They can then share some of their own concerns as well as knowledge. This mutual trust results in a dignified pregnancy, labour, delivery, and postnatal period for the woman, and hopefully a more satisfying experience for the health professionals.

Practical steps

Communicate directly with the disabled woman: even if the woman is accompanied by a non-disabled person such as an interpreter, spouse, parent or friend, address all questions to her. Maintain eye contact even if you are talking to a deaf person through an interpreter. Also try not to ignore her in situations where you are just passing by her bed or talking to other mothers. You may only be talking about the weather but the social contact is just as important for her. Remember that isolation is one of the greatest problems faced by women with disabilities in hospital, particularly when the mother has a hearing or visual impairment.

Involve her partner, whether he is able-bodied or disabled. He will be more able to support her well if he feels included and his questions and worries are satisfactorily dealt with.

Refrain from making comments that create barriers: avoid comments like 'I don't know how I'd cope if I were you' or 'I really admire your courage' or 'What happened to you, love?' Comments like this can be patronising and emphasise that you are only seeing the woman's disability, not her. Don't treat her like a child or suggest that she has been irresponsible in becoming pregnant. Having a disabling condition usually means that a couple have considered parenthood a lot more carefully than most able-bodied couples.

Avoid insensitive or offensive language: again, think of the person first and the disability second. Refer to the pregnant woman with arthritis rather than the arthritic pregnant woman or, worse, the arthritic. Avoid terms such as: afflicted with, crippled, dumb, stricken with, defective, deformed, invalid, pitiful, spastic, unfortunate. A woman who has a disability doesn't want pity or to be patronised. Using positive language helps cultivate a positive attitude in her care.

Talk in a normal tone of voice: unless you have ascertained that the woman is hard of hearing, don't raise your voice. There is sometimes a tendency to treat people with all sorts of disabilities as if they are foreign – by shouting and speaking more slowly than usual.

Learn about the woman's disability from her: if you have lived with a disability, you inevitably get to know your body well. A woman with a disability will be an expert on many aspects of it and should be consulted to aid in her hospital care and to avoid any unnecessary complications.

Provide choice: do not automatically label the disabled woman as 'high-risk' unless you have firm reason to do so. Whenever possible, she should be allowed the same choices in management and treatment as an able-bodied woman. With a little forethought, childbirth positions and breastfeeding can usually be adapted to meet the needs of a disabled woman.

Educate: explain procedures in detail and obtain feedback from the woman. As a TV producer, an oft-repeated exhortation I heard was, 'Always underestimate a viewer's knowledge but never underestimate his intelligence' – the same could be applied to medical professionals dealing with patients. Anxiety can often be removed by careful explanation of what you intend to do and why. Always explain any medical terminology that you have to use. Also, be prepared to admit when medical knowledge is lacking or insufficient so that a couple can understand the basis for your advice.

Use your contact with the disabled woman to expand her general gynaecological knowledge, for example, showing her how to examine her breasts, discussing contraception methods.

Treat her as an individual: every pregnant woman is different, disabled or not. While previous experience may give you an insight into likely problems a woman may encounter in pregnancy and with childcare, don't assume they will arise. For example, statistically, most women with spina bifida have their babies delivered by Caesarean section but that does not mean that all women with spina bifida need to have a

Caesarean. It may be more convenient for the obstetrician but it may not be so for the woman.

Refer and consult when appropriate: doctors clearly need to keep in touch with other physicians caring for the disabled woman. The obstetrician will know the woman's medical history from her GP's notes and from her, but other specialists (such as a rheumatologist or neurologist) may also need to stay involved and in contact with him during her pregnancy. The woman may also need to be referred to a physiotherapist and/or occupational therapist. Try to inform the woman of sources of support for beyond the birth too – for example, a woman with bladder incontinence may need specialist advice from a urologist after birth.

Provide a barrier-free environment whenever possible: physical barriers affect self-esteem. Most disabled women reach some degree of independence and feel most secure when they can attend to their own personal needs. It may be that a minor adaptation to your office, examining room, classroom or hospital environment can make a big difference in the woman's ability to maintain her independence. Examples are: making a service lift available to wheelchair users; ensuring that toilets and dressing rooms are wide enough to allow a wheelchair through, and that handrails are provided; providing cots that a disabled woman can easily reach herself to lift her baby in and out.

For more involved adaptations, take advice from an occupational therapist and physiotherapist. They may, for example, be able to provide toilet seat boosters for women who have difficulty in bending their knees, transfer boards to help getting on and off a bed, and so on.

A blind woman could be greatly helped by someone taking the time to orient her to a new environment. A deaf woman should be provided with satisfactory communication. Both these steps are to ensure safety as well as dignity.

Ask a disabled woman what help she needs before assisting her: here too, she is the expert. Even if she appears slow at times, she may prefer to do things for herself. Explanations must accompany any change in her routine – for example, the use of sterile technique for catheterisation while in hospital should be explained to a spinal cord injured woman since many catheterise themselves at home using a clean-touch technique. Do not move an empty wheelchair or other piece of equipment belonging to a person with a disability without asking permission first. Do not distract a guide dog when the owner is working the dog (that is, when the owner's hand is on the harness).

Take the initiative: why not try to organise a department meeting to discuss how you could provide a better service to mothers with special needs? Talk to local self-help groups for advice on specific disabilities or contact the national societies (addresses at the end of each chapter). You will find people more than willing to give you information that enables you to give better care.

And, if you find yourself working with a mother who has a disability, use the opportunity to find out more about her needs and how best to cater for them – then consider publishing the case history. There is not enough published information available when it comes to the medical and practical treatment of mothers with disabilities and you may be in a position to help on a wider level.

Impart confidence: my own research has emphasised previous American findings that medical staff attitudes are a major problem and that either abortion or adoption is too readily recommended to disabled parents. Eradicating ignorance and accepting the sexuality and parental rights of people with disabilities is the next major hurdle in the fight for equality – and your role is crucial. When a problem arises, a professional carer who says, 'Yes, that's a concern, but let's try to find a way round it' can change a frightening experience into a satisfying one.

An additional guide for antenatal teachers

As well as the above points you may find the following practical tips useful when teaching a group of pregnant women which includes anyone with a disability.

Bear in mind that the woman may be nervous of this new situation and self-conscious of her disability. If at all possible, see her separately before the first class and get to know her and her disability so you can adapt and offer additional help when appropriate. Be relaxed and friendly with her and encourage her to ask questions and express her feelings. In class, try not to make a fuss of her or draw attention to her unnecessarily.

Blind or partially sighted women: if you are teaching a group of women including a woman with seeing difficulties, remember to ask everyone to identify themselves at the start of each class and acknowledge by name any new person arriving or leaving. This enables her to get to know the rest of the class and so fulfils a vital part of group teaching. If you demonstrate any piece of equipment (such as the gas-and-oxygen mask or changing a nappy with a doll) allow her to feel the objects. Don't make a fuss about this – there is no reason why it should take more additional effort, just a bit of considerate forethought. When using an anatomical model, the blind person needs to know if the model is life-size and where on the body it fits. Explain 'up' and 'down', 'right' and 'left'. If you show a film in class, offer commentary over bits where the existing one doesn't explain what is going on.

If you hand out any printed notes in class, don't fail to give them to the blind woman – she can ask her partner or friend to read and tape them for her. You may like to suggest that she brings a tape recorder to tape part of the actual classes – mention this in private. Contact, or suggest that the woman contact, any organisations that have taped or Braille material on childbirth preparations. I give names and addresses in the specific chapter on visual impairment.

Remember that many partially sighted people can see posters or other printed materials if they are printed in large type and high-contrast colours like black on white instead of brown on beige.

As far as baby care is concerned, remember that more explicit verbal instructions may be necessary, and allow the blind woman to handle the doll that is being changed or bathed. Breastfeeding in particular may need a physical demonstration – again, offer this in private if possible. Talk about marking baby toiletries for easy recognition and discuss with the woman arrangements for getting to the hospital in an emergency.

Hearing-impaired women: first ascertain the extent of her hearing loss. Find out in advance whether the woman wishes to communicate through lip-reading, writing or sign-language and interpreter. If she chooses sign-language she may already have an interpreter, or you can arrange for one by contacting a local hearing and speech centre. Both the interpreter and the deaf person should receive a list of the childbirth-related words used in class and their definitions – in advance.

If the woman prefers to read lips, make sure that you face her when you are speaking, and that the room and you are well lit. Speak in a normal tone of voice without exaggerated movements but try to articulate words clearly. Use short, simple sentences and give her a childbirth vocabulary. When you are not understood, rephrase the sentence instead of repeating it word for word, and write down words that seem especially difficult. Even the best lip-readers can only understand 25 per cent of what is said, so do question the woman frequently to see whether she has received your information accurately.

Writing is laborious and not usually satisfactory for lengthy or in-depth communication. If you do write, use simple words and short sentences. Always address the deaf woman directly (don't ask her interpreter, 'Does she understand?'). Always approach her from the front.

Audiovisual materials can be used to communicate with the deaf, but remember that a hearing-impaired person cannot simultaneously focus on a speaker and on visuals. When you point to something, allow her time to see what it is you have indicated and to look back at you, then resume speaking. A film is fine if the soundtrack is secondary to the picture, or if an interpreter can sign along with the film.

You and the other members of the group should be aware that deaf people can miss the subtleties of language and therefore may be labelled rude or insensitive. Such labels are unfair because the misinterpreted actions are related more to the hearing impairment than to personality.

Planning for the postnatal period should include consideration of how a deaf parent will know when her baby cries. There are monitoring devices on the market which flash when the infant makes a noise.

Women with mobility impairment: some mobility-impaired people view their wheelchairs, crutches or cane as an extension of their body. Many prefer to move their wheelchairs themselves. Accordingly, consult with the mobility-impaired woman before moving her crutches or chair. Avoid leaning on the chair or resting your hands on it. If you are going to speak to her for longer than a few moments, pull up a seat or kneel on the floor to get to the same eye level as her.

References and acknowledgements

Wilma Asrael's work at the Charlotte Rehabilitation Hospital in North Carolina has been an inspiration in writing this chapter and I would like to acknowledge with gratitude her permission to use extracts from the following two articles:

Asrael, W. (1983) *Disabled Women and Childbearing: The Nurse's Role*, Nurses' Association American College of Obstetricians and Gynaecologists (NAACOG) Update Series.

Asrael, W. and Kesselman, S. (Winter 1982) 'Classes for the disabled', *Childbirth Educator*.

Further reading

Banson-Idun, A. (March 1984) 'Supporting disabled parents in the community', *Nursing Times*.

Smithers, K. (May 1986) 'Health visiting in practice: case study of a disabled mother (MS)', *Health Visitor*.

Conine, T.A., and Carty, E.A. (November 1986) 'Childbirth education for disabled parents: Psychosocial considerations', *International Journal of Childbirth Education*.

See also references in Chapter 1 and specific disability chapters in Part 2.

Part two

Preface

In Part 2, I have taken some of the more common conditions that can cause physical disability, in order to look at how they may affect, or be affected by, pregnancy and childbirth. I have chosen to look only at those which usually permit childbirth to take place without adversely affecting mother or baby and where I felt able to give information that would be useful to all women with that condition.

There is much variation in what is defined as physical disability, and while all women with, for example, asthma, diabetes or epilepsy may not regard themselves as physically disabled, after much consultation I decided that it would be helpful to include chapters on these conditions.

My definition of disability is therefore a broad one: any physical condition which restricts a person from using their body as fully and as easily as an able-bodied person. Often the restrictions are imposed by the outside world, for example, inaccessible buildings or equipment; at other times (as with hearing or visual impairments, for example) the restrictions are ones which limit access to information.

This section is NOT intended as a guide to all medical illnesses in pregnancy. It is possible to be disabled and perfectly healthy – neither being pregnant nor being disabled is an illness, and therefore the expertise for either cannot rest solely with the medical profession. Conversely, it is, of course, possible to be disabled by a medical condition such as heart disease or diabetes if the severity of the condition is such that it restricts normal life.

I hope that, whatever your disability, you will find the following accounts useful and that they will help you formulate the questions to ask – to get the information and support YOU need. I would like to stress that, for every woman, the way the disability affects you, and the way your body copes with pregnancy, is unique to you; what follows are only general points. Individual circumstances obviously cannot be predicted and that is why it is so important for professionals to look at you as an individual and to assess your situation accordingly.

The personal experiences reproduced here show up examples of the sort of problems – and, indeed, of the good practice – that a disabled woman may encounter during pregnancy and labour. One of my criteria for including them was that the pregnancies should have taken place since 1980. I hope professionals reading these will be able to use them to examine their own practices and to raise the level of awareness of the issues relating to disability.

Some of the references I include are from specialist publications and may be difficult for readers without a medical education to follow, so I have marked these with an asterisk. To follow up a particular reference, try your local library first.

Each chapter has been checked by appropriate specialists, so all the information should be correct and up-to-date at the time of writing.

Chapter seven

Arthritis

What is arthritis?

There are several forms of arthritis. The most common is *rheumatoid arthritis*, a chronic inflammation occurring throughout the body which shows up in hot, swollen, painful joints. It may appear suddenly or gradually. The condition may be mild, following an up-and-down pattern, or it may be relentlessly progressive and disabling. It may lead to deformed joints and even to their eventual destruction.

In this condition, muscle weakening and wasting can also occur above and below the joint, both resulting in varying degrees of incapacity. The small joints of the hand, the wrist, knees, and feet are the most commonly affected. In severe cases, it can involve the elbows, shoulders, hips, and ankles.

Ankylosing spondylitis is another form of arthritis which affects the spine. It affects mainly men, but women are also affected – one in five cases of AS is a woman (more than previously thought). It can lead to severe curvature of the upper spine and to a restriction in movement of the neck. Lung expansion may also be affected, leading to difficulties in breathing comfortably.

Juvenile arthritis, as its name suggests, occurs in young children. It can be treated and in 75 per cent of cases the person recovers, but with varying degrees of residual problems. The most common of these is that growth is affected and the child may become a small adult. There is no evidence that a child who has suffered juvenile arthritis will have any other form of arthritis when he or she grows up.

There are many, many other forms of rheumatic disorder (that is, affecting the musculoskeletal system) but I will concentrate on the most common, rheumatoid arthritis.

Who gets rheumatoid arthritis?

At least half a million people in Britain suffer from rheumatoid arthritis and it affects three times as many women as men.

How does it affect daily life?

Arthritis is a chronic condition and may require the sufferer to cope with pain, reduced mobility and function, tiredness and uncertainty. Uncertainty about the course of the illness and about one's ability to cope often results in anxiety and stress.

What is the cause?

Much research is in progress to see whether the cause is an infection which affects a person's immune system. There is a genetic influence on the way we handle disease and there are enough familial cases of arthritis to suggest that genetics are involved.

Will my child inherit the disease?

About one in ten women with rheumatoid arthritis have a first-degree relative (for example, mother, sister, daughter) with arthritis but there is no predicting whether your child will get the condition and, in any case, the risk is very small and should not deter you from having children.

Can it be cured?

No, but with drugs and exercise its progress can be slowed down significantly and the discomfort controlled. Some people find special diets, for example, those which are gluten-free or dairy-product free, also help alleviate the symptoms. Foods containing gluten or dairy products may aggravate the symptoms but do not cause them.

Artificial plastic joints to replace damaged arthritic ones have given many sufferers a new lease of active life.

Can a woman with RA have children?

If you want to have children and have good medical support you can probably go ahead and have them. The main consideration is how YOU will cope physically. There is no doubt that the sheer additional weight that you will have to carry during pregnancy is likely to aggravate knee, hip, and back problems and that your condition may well suffer a flare-up of the disease after the birth of the baby – just when you need to be at your fittest.

If you decide to go ahead, you should discuss the matter with your rheumatologist before actually becoming pregnant, as the drugs you are taking may be dangerous to the foetus and may need to be changed. A rheumatologist is likely to recommend that you are only on the mildest of NSAIDs (non-steroidal anti-inflammatory drugs) while trying to conceive and in pregnancy.

It is also important to avoid X-rays during the first 3 months of the pregnancy. Make sure your rheumatologist knows if you are pregnant so that these are not done.

In the long term, there is no evidence to suggest that pregnancy will have either a beneficial or a detrimental effect on the progress of your arthritis.

Will it affect fertility?

There is no medical evidence to suggest that rheumatoid arthritis affects fertility although it does seem that some women with rheumatoid arthritis take a long time to conceive.

Some drugs are known to upset the menstrual cycle, so you may need to stop taking these before trying to get pregnant. If you see your rheumatologist he will advise you about this.

Will I have to have a Caesarean?

Rheumatoid arthritis does not in itself prevent vaginal delivery unless the hip joints are affected to a degree that thighs cannot be separated comfortably or if the pelvis is too small. The latter is most likely among women who have had juvenile arthritis.

If you have had a hip replacement you are also likely to need a Caesarean section.

What are the risks of the drugs I am taking to the baby?

Ideally every pregnant woman with arthritis wants to avoid any skeletal damage, to be free from pain and to be able to carry out daily activities safely. Drugs will be a crucial factor in achieving all these goals – they will be used to relieve symptoms and to help arrest the progression of the disease. If the pregnancy is planned, you can ensure that your rheumatologist assesses and adapts your drug regime before you become pregnant.

There is no agreement about the exact dangers to the foetus of many of the drugs used to treat rheumatoid arthritis. However, the following recommendations will be borne in mind by your rheumatologist when he advises you:

1. Non-salicylate analgesics should be used because salicylates (for example, aspirin) have been associated with an interference in the bloodclotting mechanism in newborn babies, respiratory distress syndrome, and, in large amounts, with decreased birth weight and an increased stillbirth rate.

2. NSAIDs (for example, indomethacin) should be used with caution. The release of certain local hormones, known as prostaglandins, trigger the inflammation in rheumatoid arthritis and indomethacin works by suppressing the release of these – so its effects on the foetus are unclear.

3. Low doses of corticosteroids (for example, hydrocortisone) are acceptable with increases in dosage to cover the stress of labour and delivery and in anticipation of postnatal worsening. These drugs can affect the baby's output of adrenal hormones, so the newborn must be watched carefully.

4. Immuno-suppressants have not been established as safe for mother and foetus.

5. The safety of gold is unclear and should not be used unless absolutely necessary.

6. Penicillamine is often recommended for those patients who do not respond to NSAIDs but its exact mechanism is unknown and it does have a high incidence of side-effects. These affect blood and kidney function which makes it unsuitable for use during pregnancy.

How will the pregnancy affect the arthritis?

For three-quarters of all women with rheumatoid arthritis, pregnancy brings some remission of the disease, the improvement gradually developing from after the first trimester. It takes the form of a decrease in morning stiffness and joint tenderness, fewer swollen joints, an increase in grip strength, and improvement in the performance of daily activities.

However, 95 per cent of those who obtain relief experience a flare-up in the postnatal period, usually within three months of the delivery.

This still leaves a quarter of the women requiring some form of continuing treatment during pregnancy.

Anaemia

Major cardiovascular and respiratory changes occur during the course of any pregnancy. The amount of blood circulating in your body increases by 40 per cent to support the growing baby and there is a risk of iron-deficiency anaemia. Blood tests are done as routine during pregnancy and if anaemia is discovered, iron tablets are prescribed.

Women with chronic arthritis are even more vulnerable to anaemia than other pregnant women as the haemoglobin in the blood is already lower – the extra demands of the baby may make it plummet to dangerous levels unless carefully monitored. Signs of anaemia are tiredness and shortness of breath.

Breathlessness

During a normal pregnancy the space available for lung expansion to breath is substantially altered by the growing baby. The diaphragm may rise by as much as 4 cm and the circumference of your thoracic rib-cage can increase by 5–7 cm. Women with spinal arthritis may find that these alterations cause discomfort and, particularly late in pregnancy, have difficulty in breathing. Your physiotherapist should be able to advise you on ways of obtaining relief.

Any precautions during pregnancy?

The most challenging feature of pregnancy for women with rheumatoid arthritis is fatigue, particularly in the first three months of the pregnancy and then again after the baby is born. These periods are exhausting for all women but in the woman with RA they are compounded by the inflammatory process associated with the disease which can produce overwhelming fatigue.

The majority of women with RA will have already developed strategies for living as normally as possible despite the disease. Pacing and rest are the two crucial points to mention here:

Pacing: Identify which activities you can do.

Know under what circumstances and how often they can be done.

Plan the day and week accordingly.

Rest: Try to get at least two daily rest periods of 1 hour each.

Sleep 8 – 10 hours at night.

Sit to work whenever possible.

Plan to do tiring activities at intervals throughout the day.

Avoid being overtired at the end of the day.

Pay special attention to: table and chair heights;

back and seat support in chairs and cars;

bed height and mattress support.

Joint rest: This is as important as general rest, particularly because it helps to relieve pain. Working splints may be necessary. Also recommended are rest periods in specified postures – see your physiotherapist for advice on this.

Exercise: Just as frequent rest periods are needed to alleviate fatigue, exercise is needed to reduce stiffness, and to prevent muscle wasting and the loss of joint mobility. During an acute phase of the disease, appropriate exercise consists of a gentle, full range of motion exercises carried out once or twice a day just to the point of pain to help minimise stiffening up.

Otherwise, daily exercise should consist of warm-up stretching, followed by some maximal stretching exercises. The particular exercise routine for any woman should be directed by your own regular physiotherapist.

Swimming is one of the best all-round exercises for women with rheumatoid arthritis, even through the last months of the pregnancy, although over-tiredness and chilling should be avoided and strokes that could result in strain should not be used. During the postnatal period you should wait until the lochia (bleeding) has stopped before resuming swimming.

Antenatal checks: If you have trouble getting on to the examining couch, ask the midwife to assist you. Unfortunately, most hospital beds seem to be too high for most women and you may need to be lifted. If your partner can attend, it may make your checks more comfortable. If you have difficulty getting your knees apart for internal examinations, these should be done while you lie on your side.

Diet: Rheumatoid arthritis should not affect eating habits during pregnancy. If you are taking steroids they tend to increase the appetite, so you must be careful to avoid excessive weight gain. Excessive weight may cause problems for labour and delivery as well as put stress on affected joints.

Sex: If pain is the problem, some of the following suggestions might be useful: use an analgesic so that it peaks when you wish to make love; take a warm bath or shower before sex to help relieve joint stiffness; incorporate a range of motion exercises and light massage into sexual pleasuring; try a variety of positions to achieve the maximum relaxation and pleasure; have sex at a time when feeling rested.

Precautions during labour

The positions you can adopt during labour may be restricted, but often lying on the left side rather than on the back is more comfortable. Midwives are familiar with this position and may even suggest it.

Epidural anaesthetic for a woman with spinal arthritis may be impossible or inadvisable because of the difficulty in placing the needle in the spine accurately. Because of the risk of instability of the joints between the top two bones in the spine, just below the skull, special care will be needed should you need a general anaesthetic. A collar will be used to prevent throwing the head back too far, which could result in injury to the upper cervical spine.

Women with stiffness in the spine below the neck may also be difficult to intubate (that is, have tubes inserted down nose or mouth) for a general anaesthetic so an epidural may be used instead.

On the postnatal ward

Breastfeeding

The severity of your disease will determine how much medication is necessary and whether the drug levels in your breastmilk are acceptable or not. It will also determine whether you have the energy required to breastfeed and whether it is physically comfortable to do so.

Find out beforehand from your doctor (preferably your rheumatologist) about what dosages of your drugs are safe for breastfeeding.

One mother, who had decided to bottle-feed because of the stiffness in her neck and shoulder, was surprised when she was told she would have to breastfeed for a while. Apparently this was to stop the baby suffering from withdrawal symptoms as the drugs she had been taking were mildly addictive.

One new mother suggested taking your own chair into hospital as the ones in the postnatal ward tend to be very low and may be difficult to get on and off for feeding. You may also find breastfeeding easier to do while lying on your side.

Looking after yourself

Few hospital beds are comfortable either to sleep in or to get in and out of if you have stiff joints. Ask the Sister on the ward whether there are any which can be lowered electrically, or even manually controlled ones which can be left in the lowest position. Otherwise you will have to ask for help each time you want to get up, which is frustrating.

Your own duvet instead of the hospital blankets may be more comfortable, but remember that most hospital wards are kept at very warm temperatures.

The other major problem is likely to be using the bathroom – hospital baths are usually impossible to get into, and bidets are usually too low. A shower-bench may be the only feasible option, especially if your partner or other relative can come in and help you until you get home.

Also remember to take your drugs in with you – you should take anything you use routinely and give it to the Sister on admission.

Looking after baby

Start thinking about this before the baby is born. How much you will need to adapt ways of baby care will obviously depend on the severity with which the disease affects you. The Under-35 Group of Arthritis Care runs a counselling network to enable new mothers to benefit from the experiences of other mothers with arthritis. An occupational therapist may be able to provide useful tips too.

Rheumatoid arthritis: case history 1

I was 26 when my husband and I began to think about starting a family. I had had rheumatoid arthritis for 5 years but was able to walk and lead an active life and held a job as a receptionist at a large firm of solicitors in Bradford. I was quite worried about how I would cope with pregnancy and, as I had had no contact with young children, I wondered how I would cope with looking after a child.

We were both also concerned about whether the child would be affected by the disease and so asked our GP to refer us to a genetic counsellor. He refused initially but we did eventually get to see one of the country's leading counsellors.

We found the genetic counsellor both kind and helpful. He advised us against having a child more for my sake than for the child's. In coming to this, he asked us to consider the difficulties I would have looking after a baby, coping with lack of sleep and probably a deterioration in my condition in the long-term. As for the baby, there was a very small risk, particularly if a girl, that it might develop the disease.

We came home to think about his advice. I very much wanted children and knew that Alan wanted them even more and would be very disappointed if we were not able to have any. I was dismayed at the prospect of my arthritis getting worse as a result of having children but then wondered whether it might do so anyway. We decided to go ahead.

I had no menstrual cycle because of the painkiller I had been taking so had to have fertility drugs. I became pregnant within a month and booked in at a nearby 12-bed GP unit rather than the big Clarendon wing in Leeds. I felt that they would be able to give me more personal attention being a smaller set-up. At first there was a reluctance to take me as the GP unit could not provide as great a range of pain relief.

This didn't put me off. I had been told that I wouldn't be able to have an epidural because of my spine; I didn't think I could have pethidine because I can't handle alcohol and I had heard that this meant that you should avoid pethidine. (Both of these assumptions I later found out to be incorrect.) I am used to coping with intense pain so I thought I would manage somehow.

I found my health improved and the arthritis decreased all through the second trimester, but the last few months were exhausting. The midwives who supervised me antenatally were very helpful and I was told to bring into hospital anything that would make my stay more comfortable.

I never did any exercise before my pregnancy and had never met a physiotherapist so had no idea what I could do. My back and knees suffered badly with the increasing burden of the baby. I attended an NCT class for a while, which I enjoyed, but was nearly put off by the scatter cushions on the floor ('Haven't you got a chair?!'). I found the advice regarding delivery positions irrelevant and so ignored it. But I did find the breathing techniques and relaxation exercises useful and have remained friends with some of the women I met in the class.

My health visitor did not have much specific advice to help me with the disability but was able to give some general advice on baby care. I also received a lot of useful advice about what to buy from the Arthritis Care Under-35 Group.

The birth day was 10 days late but went like a dream. It was all over in 2 hours and the midwives were wonderful. I was told to get comfortable and they would deliver me in whatever position that was – in my case, lying on my left side.

Our daughter Katie was born at 12 noon. It was a wonderful moment – we were both in tears for half an hour, just looking at her!

I had needed no form of pain relief as it was over so quickly, but I did need stitches which the midwives performed skilfully while I continued to lie on my side.

Back on the ward with my husband, I was in a daze of happiness and don't recall any particular difficulties. My only criticism was that no lunch was booked for me so I didn't get to eat until 5.30 pm – which was dangerous as I have to take my drugs with food. Next time round I took food supplies with me.

I only stayed in the hospital for 48 hours as I have a waterbed at home and I had help organised, so the midwives agreed I would be better off there.

I had decided to breastfeed and managed well by using a pillow on my lap to raise the baby. The problems came when she was 7 months old and I had a flare-up in the disease which meant taking anti-inflammatory drugs that got into the breast milk. I had to stop breast-feeding earlier than I had intended.

I found caring for the baby hard work, and feel I hurt my back carrying her around and up and down stairs. Once she was mobile I was restricted to one room that had been made baby-proof. When Katie was $2^{1/2}$, I was forced to take to a wheelchair to get around outside.

An occupational therapist came to our home and arranged all sorts of adaptations to be done, entirely at the expense of the local council.

A year later I embarked on a second pregnancy, my condition much deteriorated, and unfortunately had no remission during the 9 months at all. (I wonder whether the fact I was carrying a boy that time made a difference.) I had the baby at the GP unit again and the labour was even quicker (less than an hour) and I was back home the same day.

Being restricted by a wheelchair out of doors does limit my ability to *get around much more and the main effect of this is isolation. I don't get to meet other mums at the school gates or get out to mother-and-toddler groups because they are in inaccessible places. This does worry me because in the past I used to travel quite a bit to counsel other women with arthritis for Arthritis Care Under-35 Group of which I was a very active member.*

I now have a home-help for a few hours each week and my husband continues to share the work of looking after the children, taking over the bathing and feeding when he comes home from work. I have taken advantage of an IT offer of a home computing course which I enjoy very much and would like to put to use in the future.

Tom is now 1 and Katie 5, and there is no doubt that I feel less able than before I took on motherhood. Katie has no hang-ups about my disability and has met many other wheelchair users at a local disabled club so doesn't feel that her mother is any way less of a mother. I could cite many examples of Katie's independence and self-assurance and have no regrets about my decision to have children. It's either in your soul or it isn't and in my case the desire to have children and the conviction that we could be good parents over-ruled the worries about my arthritis.

Rheumatoid arthritis: case history 2

I have suffered from rheumatoid arthritis since I was 6 years old. I am now 26 and my main worries before becoming pregnant were: would I be able to carry the baby full term, would the extra weight cause further damage to my hips, spine, and knees and would I be able to give birth normally?

I consulted my rheumatologist (whom I thought the best person as he knew more about my condition than my own GP) who sent me for several tests. The tests included X-rays on my hips, an ECG, and my kidneys were tested to make sure they were functioning properly. I also had a chat with a gynaecologist. Both were very understanding and my rheumatologist said he could see no reason why I should not have a baby.

So we went ahead. I had been told that because I had arthritis it might take quite some time to conceive but in fact I became pregnant in a few weeks.

I read a few books on pregnancy from the library but there is no particular one I would recommend – they all seemed to offer the same information. My GP was very good at putting my mind at rest if I had any worries.

The only problems I had during pregnancy were a urinary tract infection (common in pregnancy, I was told) and high blood pressure. For the infection I was given a course of antibiotics. My blood pressure was monitored closely in the final trimester by a district midwife but, despite rest, it didn't come down, so I was admitted to hospital at 36 weeks.

I had no problems that I would attribute to the arthritis. Surprisingly, I didn't suffer from the extra weight I was putting on to my joints. I did tire towards the end but I think most pregnant women do.

I did attend the antenatal clinic at the hospital and had no problems with either access or the staff. They allowed my husband to come into the examination room with me so that he could help me with undressing/dressing and getting on and off the bed.

I also attended the first three antenatal classes but missed the last five because of going into hospital early. The few I did attend were quite useful, although there was no attempt to adapt to my special needs.

I was given useful advice about exercise, breathing and diet. I did not follow the exercise routine for fear of damaging my joints and thought the breathing techniques unnecessary as I was to have a Caesarean.

With regard to equipment, etc., I was given additional useful advice by the occupational therapist to help prepare for the baby.

The birth was by Caesarean as I had been told that I had only restricted movement in my hips. I felt the Caesarean was managed very well. There was a slight problem inserting the needle into my spine for the epidural. This was because of the arthritis and the damage it had caused, but it did eventually take effect.

I was treated very well by both doctors and midwives: they all seemed very sympathetic towards my disability.

Because I had an epidural I was awake throughout the Caesarean and my husband stayed with me all the time. I held my baby almost immediately after the birth. The moment I first held my son I felt overwhelming joy. I couldn't believe he was mine, I couldn't stop crying. I felt so complete.

On the postnatal ward I found it very difficult to get any rest as the beds were so uncomfortable. I suffered more with the arthritis because of that. Also, none of the beds were of the right height to enable me to get in and out myself, so I had to call a nurse every time I had to attend the baby, go to the toilet, etc. The low chairs were also a problem, but

I was allowed to bring a higher chair of my own into hospital. Once I was on my feet there was no problem. My husband was allowed to come daily to help with showering.

I didn't have too much trouble handling my baby except when breastfeeding. I went home 6 days after having him. The first 3 or 4 weeks were the most frightening. I was so worried that I wasn't doing everything by the book and that something would happen to the baby. However, things soon settled down and I got into my own routine. I looked after baby in the way I felt right and things became a lot easier.

I had no extra help at home. Fortunately my husband is at home a lot so between the two of us we managed very well and didn't really need any outside help. We found looking after the baby fine – but doing the housework as well was rather difficult!

On reflection, the only thing I would have done differently was to have bottle fed and not breastfed the baby. I found it very difficult breastfeeding because my arms are so badly affected by the arthritis, making them ache. I also found it very hard to manoeuvre the baby into position as I have limited movement in my elbows. The other piece of advice I would offer first-time mothers is to take any help that is offered. At first you feel you will be able to manage yourself, but you soon realise it isn't that easy.

Rheumatoid arthritis: case history 3

I have had rheumatoid arthritis for 11 years and my disability is mild – slight damage to hand, elbow and knee joints. My daughter (age 3) was unplanned but I am now trying for another baby.

My worries are: is RA hereditary – no one seems sure – and how will I look after one child who is quite helpful when she is in the mood, as well as a helpless baby?

I told my GP and rheumatologist that I wanted another baby and waited for them to throw up their hands in horror and say, 'What on earth are you thinking of, woman!'

I had very mixed feelings about wanting another child. I do want one, desperately, but at the same time I feel very guilty about that want. No one has suggested there may be a problem but I do not feel reassured.

When I was pregnant with my daughter, I read everything and anything but did not find much that was relevant to me.

I attended the hospital antenatal clinics but because the pregnancy had been unplanned I was taking some quite risky drugs in the early weeks (penicillamine). Otherwise the only problems were tiredness (possibly due to anaemia which is common in RA) and backache after the 6th month.

The only specific advice I got was from the Arthritis Care Under-35 Group, the midwives were not able to provide any specific help antenatally.

I didn't attend antenatal classes as my daughter was a few weeks premature – a bit of a surprise all round. It was only when we booked into hospital that things started to go wrong – until then I had had a relatively straightforward pregnancy, although I had no remission.

When we arrived at the hospital with my contractions coming thick and fast, we were met by a doctor (I hadn't met him before) and told that I would be put on a drip to 'see what happens'. It was only after I'd asked for the third time that I was told it was because I might become dehydrated. My daughter was born within the hour with panic all round, and me not feeling in control at all.

As soon as she was born, they took her away to be washed while I was given some stitches – then we were wheeled into a side room so I didn't actually get to hold her for some time – I can't even remember when the first time was. My husband felt very out of it from the moment we arrived at the hospital – no one seemed to think it had anything to do with him.

I was treated throughout the labour as a problem. Straight after the birth I was told to take 50 mg of steroids. I'd already been given a 100-mg steroid injection during labour, which I had expected. I had agreed with my rheumatologist beforehand that I would double whatever dose I had got down to while I was pregnant. Eventually they phoned the registrar and he agreed with me. After that, all my tablets were returned to me and I was left to manage the RA on my own.

I was told (wrongly) I wouldn't be able to breastfeed because of the steroids, so someone would sit by me while I bottle-fed her, or worse, she would be taken from me and fed by someone else. I was never given a satisfactory reason for this. I felt terribly possessive and the RA had become more painful too as the steroid injection wore off. The bidets were too low and getting in or out of the bath was out of the question – I was glad to return home after 3 days.

My mother came to help look after us when we came home which was very helpful in getting us back into some sort of a normal life.

Since having my daughter my RA has not deteriorated. I actually feel much better since I have been on a dairy- and wheat-free diet and only get bad flare-ups when I eat the wrong things.

My advice to other women with RA is to talk to mothers who have been through it. Also, plan ahead for what help you can realistically expect. My husband is willing now to help but is usually not much use because he doesn't have much to do with the baby from day to day while at work. My mum has been my salvation and it's only because of her that I am contemplating going through it again.

Contacts

Arthritis Care: Under-35 Group
29 Darrell Close
Chelmsford
Essex CM1 4EL
Tel. 0245 358519

Will put you in touch with other mothers and advise on equipment purchase, etc.

Ankylosing Spondylitis Society
6 Grosvenor Crescent
London SW1X 7ER
Tel. 071-235 9585

Can provide information about pregnancy.

References

* Ansell, B. (ed.) (September 1988) 'Review of pregnancy and arthritis research', *Clinical and Experimental Rheumatology*.

* Carty, E., Conine, T. A., and Wood-Johnson, F. (November 1986) 'Rheumatoid arthritis and pregnancy', *Midwives Chronicle and Nursing Notes*.

* Carty, E., Conine, T. A., and Wood-Johnson, F. (1987) 'Nature and source of information received by primiparas with rheumatoid arthritis on preventative maternal and child care', *Canadian Journal of Public Health* 78 (6):393–7.

Hamilton, C. (Spring 1986) 'Coping with children when you have rheumatoid arthritis', *Arthritis Research Today*.

Harris, C. J. (1985) 'Pregnancy can offer a welcome reprieve from chronic inflammation of arthritis', *American Journal of Nursing* 85:415–17.

Khaligh, N. and Wood, P. H. N. (September 1986) *Arthritis and Rheumatism in the Eighties – a report on the burden of suffering from arthritis and rheumatism and the availability of facilities for treatment and relief*, Arthritis Research Council.

(* Publications that may prove difficult for readers without a medical education to follow.)

Further reading

Ehrlich, G. E. (1982) 'Sexual Problems of the Arthritic', in Comfort, A. (ed.) *Sexual Consequences of Disability*, Stickley.

Lorig, K. and Fries, J. (1983) *The Arthritis Helpbook*, Souvenir Press.

Arthritis and Rheumatism Council (1987) *Arthritis: Sexual Aspects and Parenthood*. Booklet available from:

Arthritis and Rheumatism Council
41 Eagle Street
London WC1R 4AR
Tel. 071-405 8572

Chapter eight

Parenting with artificial limbs

There are usually no medical problems associated with pregnancy for those women who have artificial limbs but there may be a few practical ones. The following two accounts may illustrate some of these.

Case history 1

I am a congenital amputee and have an artificial left arm. It is not due to a genetic abnormality so I was not offered genetic counselling, but I was concerned as the reason for my disability had never been established, and so I obviously felt specialist advice might have been able to reassure me that there was no risk to the baby.

I have had two children and, on the whole, I had good pregnancies with only a few problems. The first problem was caused by my prosthesis. As I put on weight it became tighter, and as it was summertime, I came up in a nasty rash too. I had previously only encountered this on hot holidays. Another thing I had to be vigilant about was that as I grew larger, my centre of gravity shifted, and my balance – which can be a bit erratic anyway – got worse and the tendency to trip got greater.

The medical care I had was reasonable. The GP was sympathetic and supportive throughout but I had a few problems in hospital in my first pregnancy. I was offered an elective Caesarean section which my GP could not understand as there was nothing in my obstetric history to warrant this. Further inquiry revealed that this was because I was thought to have an artificial foot, but even then we were given no satisfactory explanation as to why a Caesarean would have been necessary. I had seen the consultant twice and he had somehow failed to recognise that it was my arm which was artificial not my foot. I found this both hilarious and extremely worrying.

My other problem relates to a remark made by the surgery nurse. At my first antenatal visit I was greeted with 'How do you think you'll manage a baby?' The nurse was extremely derisory and undermined my confidence. So much for shared care!

I attended classes during my first pregnancy but I did not find them particularly helpful apart from being given the opportunity to meet other mums. They made no attempt to cater for my special needs and, at that stage, I had no idea of what my special needs might be anyway. My life is totally adaptive so I knew I would have to have a time of trial and error. The health visitor who saw me antenatally was the same – she advised me generally but did not attempt to gear what she said to my disability.

Both labours were straightforward and I needed no pain relief or special attention. The midwives I had during labour were excellent and I felt an immediate rapport with them. I saw doctors so briefly that I feel their treatment of me just doesn't matter. However, my arrival on the ward and treatment by the midwives there is a different story.

I rarely saw the same midwives twice and felt ignored much of the time. I find it difficult to judge how true this was because of my state of mind at that time. I felt very vulnerable. After two days I was transferred to a smaller unit and relaxed in the totally different atmosphere. My only bad moment was when I was ordered to bathe my son and felt obliged to comply – I nearly drowned him because I was feeling a bit shaky at the time.

On the second occasion I was in the local GP unit and it was a much more relaxed atmosphere from the start. Unfortunately my best artificial limb broke the week before I gave birth. Therefore I needed more help than I had anticipated. I felt bad because I had to keep asking for help. I was offered a separate room which I declined as I would have felt too isolated.

Looking back, I felt that hospital was the right place for me to have my baby, but I felt like a fish out of water in the unfamiliar surroundings. At home I work on the floor because I feel my baby is safer there. I did not feel able to do this in hospital.

Initially I had problems with all aspects of child care. It had to be a case of trial and error but I managed this quite easily and successfully. It is very difficult for anyone who does not have my disability to advise me. I don't do anything like a 'normal' person. Luckily, I have found my children to be very resilient.

I went home after a week on both occasions. I find it very difficult to express my feelings about being at home, totally responsible for the welfare of a tiny infant. We moved house when my son was 4 months old. It was a very bad winter and I ended up feeling very depressed.

I had my mother come to stay for a week on both occasions but it was not a success because I was very emotional. I think I would have been better off with good impartial help.

Perhaps the best advice I could offer someone with a similar disability is to contact someone like me. Ultimately each individual has to do things her own way, but to talk in practical terms with someone in the same boat can cut corners, save time, and improve confidence. It is very easy to let minor problems add up! I know that when I once jabbed my baby son with a nappy pin, I felt as if my world had ended! Second pregnancies and babyhoods are easier, but how you cope still depends very much on the personality of the baby.

Case history 2

I lost both legs in a farming accident when I was 2 and get around on crutches.

My husband and I had not planned on having a family but, despite taking precautions, I became pregnant. It was a bit of a surprise but I started reading and trying to get information about pregnancy straightaway. I came across nothing which mentioned disability and my GP was not able to help much either as she had not come across a disabled pregnant woman before so didn't know how to react at all.

I had an uncomfortable pregnancy with a lot of nausea and backache but no one could say any more than 'It's all part of being pregnant'. I carried my baby on my left side all through the pregnancy which made me look very odd.

I attended antenatal clinics at the local hospital and had no problems with access. One midwife made such a fuss over me that she made me feel embarrassed to be there. The consultant just said he had never in all his years had a patient as disabled as me, which didn't exactly help boost my confidence.

I went to one antenatal class and was made to feel so outcast that I never went back. There was no attempt to meet my special needs. Generally, I was given no advice about exercise or diet other than what

I read myself. I would have liked to know what exercises I was capable of.

My health visitor was quite helpful in her own way but unfortunately I only met her once before the baby was born.

Four weeks in advance of the birth I went into hospital as it was getting more and more difficult to get around on crutches and also my blood pressure was going up.

I had a Caesarean as I was told that my pelvis was not only too small to take the baby's head but also out of line due to my disability. The baby's head never descended into the pelvis right up to the morning of the Caesarean.

Most of the staff treated us well. The junior doctor in particular did try to understand the difficulties I had. On the antenatal ward the midwives were very friendly. The trainees were the best of all as they found time to just come over and talk, to learn about disabled people and pregnancy.

After the Caesarean (under a general anaesthetic) I held the baby as soon as I came round. My emotions were of delight, excitement and relief that it was over. My husband stayed in the next room while the Caesarean was carried out and he got a bit frustrated at a lot of his worries not being answered by the doctors.

I hated being in hospital as we were only allowed 2 hours visiting per day. As we lived 3 hours away from the hospital it meant that my husband was not able to come in the afternoon, go home, and then come back in the evening. It put quite a lot of strain on him. I understand that visiting hours in hospital are much more flexible now, but at the time it did not occur to us that, because of my disability, we could have asked for longer visiting anyway.

I had a few problems getting around on crutches and the nurses were very wary of me moving around unaccompanied. I had a relatively easy time learning to handle my daughter but had no advice at all on breastfeeding until it was too late. I had to stop because I was told I had infections in my breast. I did get advice on how to bath her and how to hold her head while washing her.

I went home after 8 days and felt very tired and angry that, as a result of an infection of my stitches, it took a lot longer for me to get up and about.

The only help I had at home was from my husband who was great and very supportive. I would not have got through it without him. Later on I got a home-help for 4 hours per week.

So what would I do different next time? I would plan ahead more in terms of breastfeeding, staying in hospital. I would insist that the doctors and midwives told me what I wanted to know when I wanted to know it. I would enjoy my pregnancy to the full and, most of all, enjoy the baby when it arrives as it is a great blessing.

Further reading

Washam, V. (1973) *The One-hander's Book: A Basic Guide to Activities of Daily Living*, New York: The John Day Company

Chapter nine

Asthma

Nowadays, most women with asthma are not disabled by it, but I include this chapter for those women for whom pregnancy is a concern.

What is asthma?

Asthma is a lung disease where the smaller airways in the lungs intermittently narrow, causing wheezy breathing. There are different forms of asthma but all share these characteristics.

Who gets it?

It can affect a person of any age (although few babies get it) and in young children often disappears by the teenage years. Amongst adults it is thought to affect as many as 4 in 100 people in this country.

How does it affect daily life?

During an asthmatic attack a person feels short of breath and struggles to breathe out. If the attack is particularly severe the function of the lungs may be affected and the person may start turning blue (a sign that not enough oxygen is reaching the blood).

However, these attacks are occasional and during the rest of the time the only way it affects life is that the person has to avoid anything which she knows might bring on an attack. This may include certain forms of exercise (such as sprinting) which require sudden vigorous breathing, stressful situations and any known allergens.

What is the cause?

The narrowing of the airways is the result of inflammation which causes swelling of their inner linings and excess production of thick, sticky phlegm. To aggravate this further, during an attack, as the person tries to breathe out the air pressure builds up in the chest and compresses the airways even more.

There are two types of true asthma – atopic and non-atopic. Atopic asthma (most common in children) is often linked to specific allergens such as house-dust or pollen.

Non-atopic is the type of asthma that tends to appear in adulthood and is not linked to allergens. When an attack comes it tends to last longer and is often more serious. Often non-atopic asthma becomes chronic (long-lasting) and may need continuous treatment with powerful drugs.

Can it be cured?

Drug treatment is often successful at reducing the frequency and severity of attacks but may not cure the disease completely.

Can a woman who has asthma have children?

Yes, there is no physical reason why the asthma should prevent you having a baby.

Will it affect fertility?

No.

Drugs and risk to baby before conception

It is important to discuss the drugs you are taking with your GP prior to trying to become pregnant. Most drugs used for treating asthma are thought to be harmless, with the possible exception of steroids taken as tablets rather than inhaled. Again, discussion with your doctor should put your mind at rest about these.

The other group of drugs that you might take are antibiotics for chest infections. Most are safe but tetracycline is to be avoided as it can cause permanent discoloration of the baby's teeth.

Will the child get asthma?

If your asthma is atopic (caused by allergens), there is a 1 in 10 chance that your child will inherit some form of allergic condition such as eczema or asthma. If both parents have atopic asthma, then the risk goes up to about 1 in 3.

If your asthma is non-atopic the risk is less clear.

How will the pregnancy affect the asthma?

Asthma is a variable condition which affects every person differently, pregnant or not, so it is difficult to predict what course it will take during your pregnancy.

The current belief is that there should be no harmful effect in terms of the frequency or severity of your attacks either during your pregnancy or in the longer term. For a few women with very severe asthma, the added strain of carrying a growing baby may prove difficult to cope with – but this is very rare.

Labour

Many women worry about having an attack during labour but in fact this is extremely unlikely. During labour your body is producing extra cortisone and adrenalin, so naturally protecting you from an attack.

Pain relief

Make sure the doctors and midwives around you know that you suffer from asthma, but pethidine, epidural anaesthesia and Entonox are all considered safe for women with asthma.

Breastfeeding

Neither asthma nor the drugs used to treat it should prevent a woman from breastfeeding.

Looking after baby

Asthma should not pose any specific problems in one's ability to look after a baby.

Contacts

Asthma Research Council
300 Upper Street
London N1 2XX
Tel. 071-226 2260

Asthma Society and Friends of the Asthma Research Council
St Thomas's Hospital
Lambeth Palace Road
London SE1 7EH
Tel. 071-261 0110

References

Sinclair, C. (1987) *Answers to Asthma*, Optima.

Chamberlain, G. and Lumley, J. (1986) *Pre-pregnancy Care*, John Wiley.

Chapter ten

Cerebral palsy

What is cerebral palsy?

Cerebral palsy is a rather vague term which means that a developing baby has suffered brain damage either before, during or immediately after birth. Exactly which part of the brain has been damaged will determine how it affects the intelligence and functions of the person with cerebral palsy: there is an enormous variation in effects.

It is crucial for anyone providing antenatal care to a woman with cerebral palsy to ask her and her partner about the extent of her disability – don't rush to conclusions, particularly about intelligence.

How many people are affected?

There are still no accurate figures available as to the number of people in the UK with cerebral palsy. The only relevant figures are that an estimated 2.5 per 1000 babies born are affected by cerebral palsy.

How does it affect daily life?

Traditionally, cerebral palsy has been divided into two major groups: spastic and athetoid. The possible physical effects on daily life are as follows:

Spasticity: Muscle spasms.
Bowel and bladder functions affected.
Poor sight.
Poor speech.
Intelligence often below what is considered normal.

Athetosis: Movements which eventually reach their target but tend to
overshoot the mark and deviate from their fixed course.
Very exaggerated movements, sometimes of the whole body, but
especially of the face, which are also present when the action is
deliberate.
Speech disturbances which are more or less serious caused by a poor
coordination of all the organs and muscles involved in speech.
Poor ability and, often, inability to walk.
Bladder and bowel control may be affected. Often hearing is
impaired.
Although sex may be difficult, the sexual organs are not directly
affected by the cerebral palsy.
Intelligence is usually unaffected.

All the above effects may seem very drastic to a person without cerebral
palsy, but it should be remembered that often the attitudes of society
have the greatest effect on daily life for people with cerebral palsy. This,
combined with the fact that many are brought up in special schools and
kept separate from other young people, may cause isolation in
adulthood. It is often a problem to find a partner and then pursue the path
to marriage and children. However, many couples with cerebral palsy
have successfully had and brought up children.

Can it be cured?

No, but the condition itself is unlikely to deteriorate – it is not an illness.

Can a woman with CP have children?

In principle, yes, in most cases. How comfortable or easy it will be to
carry a growing baby depends on the severity of the disability.

Will it affect fertility?

No.

What is the risk to the baby?

Cerebral palsy is rarely inherited, so the risk of having a child with
cerebral palsy is not significantly different from that run by any mother,
with good medical care.

Will I have to have a Caesarean?

The most important consideration should obviously be to look at you as an individual and to assess your body's capability of delivering a baby vaginally. The possible reasons you may need a Caesarean section are: pelvic deformity and/or involuntary spasms of a degree that might interfere with a vaginal delivery. The pain of contractions may set off such spasms.

Special care during pregnancy

If you use a wheelchair, exercises which encourage good circulation are important. If bladder and/or bowel control is affected, there is a need to pay extra care during pregnancy as infections and constipation may become more of a problem. Painful muscle spasms may increase and need to be treated with appropriate medication.

Labour

Unfortunately, there is not much documented information about particular challenges during labour for women with cerebral palsy because Caesarean sections tend to be the norm.

Breastfeeding

There is usually no reason why a woman with cerebral palsy should not be able to breastfeed but it may be difficult or uncomfortable to feed the baby while holding him in your arms. Alternative positions, such as lying down beside the baby, should be tried if this is the case.

Cerebral palsy: a case history

Theresa has two children aged 4 and 2 and is expecting her third shortly. Her mother had a tilted pelvis which caused a long, drawn-out labour of several days. This is thought to have caused Theresa's cerebral palsy. Her coordination and speech are affected due to involuntary muscle movements. She uses a wheelchair and she finds it difficult to hold things but her intelligence is unaffected.

She met her husband John at a party 7 years ago. He is able-bodied and works in a local engineering business within a few minutes' walk of their home. He takes a very active role in sharing parenting and housework and the company he works for allows him enough flexibility to be able to do so.

Both John and Theresa wanted and expected to have children right from the start and were somewhat taken aback by the lack of support they were given, particularly during Theresa's first pregnancy. Access difficulties apart, attitudes of doctors and nurses were the main problem. Theresa was treated as a naughty, irresponsible child and repeatedly advised to have an abortion. Once she was into her pregnancy, the doctors and midwives tended to address their questions to John, as if she were incapable of understanding herself. When she was out shopping, people would stare at her bump disapprovingly, and even close friends and family expressed surprise.

The most frightening physical problem arising from her disability happened early on in her first pregnancy. While resting in bed one day she awoke to find her whole body had gone completely rigid. It was hours before she could manipulate her fingers enough to call the hospital. She had never experienced such muscle spasms before and later learned that they can be brought on by pregnancy. Her nightmare continued for 3 days while anti-spasmodic drugs were checked for safety in pregnancy. During her current pregnancy she has also needed anti-spasmodic drugs which she hates taking as they also have a depressant effect. She says her moods swing violently and she often gets very weepy and needs more practical support from John than usual.

All three of her births will have been by Caesarean but it is only in the present pregnancy that she has been told the reason: her pelvis is out of alignment like her mother's. She regards her stay in hospital as an ordeal to be survived as her experiences each time have been less than happy. The main problems emerged at the first birth.

She was largely ignored and felt her confidence continually being undermined. The bed and bath were impossible for her to get in and out of; surfaces designed for bathing and changing baby were out of her reach. As soon as she came home and was able to do things as they suited her she was fine and the baby thrived.

John and Theresa live in a two-bedroom bungalow on an estate where they are known and have friends. The nursery that her daughter attends is a 5-minute wheelchair ride away and since Theresa has had her electric wheelchair she can take her to nursery herself and meet the other mums at the school gates. Both the children are happy and independent. A regular home-help comes for a couple of hours each day to do some of the housework but otherwise they manage largely on their own.

Like many disabled mothers, Theresa feels that she missed out on a lot of support and friendships because NCT classes and mother-and-toddler groups are held in inaccessible places. She is a resourceful and confident woman who does not see herself as someone to be pitied but as someone who is entitled to the same treatment as any other new mother.

Contacts

The Spastic Society
12 Park Crescent
London NW1
Tel. 071-636 5020

The Spastic Society can put you in touch with other parents with cerebral palsy.

References

McCullough, A. M. (1984) 'Pregnancy in a patient with cerebral palsy', *Journal of Obstetrics and Gynaecology* 5(1):39–40.

McCullough, A. M. (November 1985) 'Problems of female sexuality and pregnancy in the female with cerebral palsy', *Journal of Maternity and Child Health* 10(11):336–8.

Further reading

Spastic Society (1978) *Sex for Young People with Spina Bifida and Cerebral Palsy*. Booklet available from The Spastic Society.

—— (March 1988) 'Disabled Parents CAN Cope', in *Disability Now*. Available from The Spastic Society.

Chapter eleven

Diabetes

The vast majority of people with diabetes nowadays can lead active, able-bodied lives, thanks to better insulin control. The disabling complications of diabetes such as blindness or amputation are much less common now because of better physical care so it is, thankfully, no longer the disabling condition it used to be. However, it remains very important to take special care in pregnancy, so I include this chapter for the benefit of the many women for whom it may be a worry and also for health professionals who may not have a wide experience of looking after pregnant women with diabetes.

What is diabetes?

Diabetes mellitus is a condition in which the body cannot properly use sugar and carbohydrates from the diet. It occurs because the pancreas is not producing enough of the hormone insulin which is needed to do this.

How many people are affected?

Diabetes is thought to affect 2 per cent of the population – about 600,000 people in the UK alone have been diagnosed as having it, and it is estimated that there are about the same number who have not been diagnosed. Women and men are equally likely to get diabetes and it can begin at any age.

It is estimated that 1 in 1000 women having babies are insulin-dependent diabetics. Between 2 and 4 in 100 women develop diabetes during pregnancy but this usually disappears after the baby is born. Urine and blood tests are designed to detect this type of diabetes so care can be taken during the pregnancy, and the treatment is different to that given to women with insulin-dependent diabetes.

How does it affect daily life?

Diet control and insulin injections are necessary to control diabetes, but most women with diabetes can lead normal lives. People on insulin experience symptoms of low blood sugar (hypoglycaemia) at times, due to excess insulin, and they need to take sugar quickly to cut short the attack.

Symptoms of hypoglycaemia include faintness, sweating, unsteadiness, and odd behaviour – this may be mistaken for drunkenness. The danger for a person with diabetes is that a hypoglycaemic attack that goes unchecked may lead to a coma. Luckily most people with diabetes recognise the symptoms at the onset of a 'hypo' and know how to take action immediately.

What is the cause?

The cause of diabetes is still not fully understood.

Can it be cured?

No, but nowadays it can be very well controlled in the majority of instances so that the complications previously associated with it (kidney failure, blindness, gangrene) can be reduced. Most women of child-bearing age with diabetes are likely to be controlling it with insulin. Older people use tablets and diet to control the disease.

Can a woman who is diabetic have children?

In the majority of cases, yes. The only exception may be if you have had longstanding diabetes with raised blood pressure and kidney problems or heart disease – the risk to both you and the baby will then be far greater. Discussion with your specialist should help you decide whether the risk is one which you wish to take.

Will it affect fertility?

No, unless the diabetes is not well controlled. If your periods are irregular, it is important to keep an accurate record of them so that it is possible to work out when conception took place.

113

How important is pre-pregnancy counselling?

Pre-pregnancy counselling is now often offered to women with diabetes as measures can be taken before conception to improve the chances of a healthy baby – so do accept it if it is available.

The preventative measures include taking tight control of your blood sugar level immediately before and during pregnancy. This would involve testing blood frequently each day, following a strictly regular meal pattern and carefully planning insulin intake.

What is the risk to the baby?

The risk that the baby may be born with diabetes or develop it is only slightly increased if the mother has diabetes. If both parents have it then the chances that their child will have diabetes is thought to be 1 in 10. Having said that, it is still not clearly understood how and why diabetes is passed on and this should not be a deterrent to having children.

In the past, a very large proportion of babies born to women with diabetes died or were born with some deformity. Thanks to better antenatal care and better management of diabetes this risk is now very much reduced.

A woman with diabetes is more likely to give birth to a baby with congenital abnormalities (1 in 10) than a non-diabetic mother (1 in 40). These figures are for serious and fatal abnormalities such as spina bifida, holes in the heart or absent kidneys. However, studies have shown that if a woman's diabetes is very closely monitored and controlled before and during pregnancy, the chances of having a child with such congenital deformities are no greater than for a non-diabetic woman.

Another major problem in the past has been that diabetic women, being more prone to having larger babies, often had to be induced at 37/38 weeks. Better insulin control has meant that this is not now always the case. The other risk is that diabetes can affect the blood flow to the placenta and possibly lead to undernourishment of the baby. Frequent ultrasound scans throughout the pregnancy will help monitor the baby's growth.

How will the pregnancy affect the diabetes?

The demands of the growing baby will mean that your insulin requirements are greater, sometimes nearly double. As soon as the baby is delivered, however, your insulin requirement will return to the pre-pregnancy level.

Hypoglycaemic reactions in early pregnancy

You are likely to have more hypos in early pregnancy for two reasons. One is because you are maintaining tight control on your blood sugar levels. Second, hormonal changes make you more prone to hypos in this period. It is important to warn your friends and family and those at work and to make sure they know how to treat you if a hypo occurs. Be careful, too, when setting out to drive any great distance.

There is also no evidence to suggest that having a hypo in pregnancy will damage the child.

Vomiting in early pregnancy

While the foetus is apparently little affected by hypoglycaemic attacks in pregnancy, it is very vulnerable to ketones. Ketones may be produced if you have high blood sugar, if you are ill for any reason, or if you vomit. You will probably have been shown how to test for ketones already and it is important to do this, particularly if you have vomiting attacks in pregnancy. You may be prescribed anti-vomiting drugs and you will also be advised of drinks that you should take after vomiting to replace the carbohydrate that you have lost (see Table 11.1).

If you discover you are producing ketones or vomiting excessively, you may be admitted to hospital for a while to monitor the baby's health.

Table 11.1 Examples of drinks recommended to be taken by pregnant women with diabetes after vomiting

The following contain 10 g carbohydrate. Take whichever you find least nauseating:

1. 10 g (2 rounded teaspoons) glucose or sugar dissolved in weak tea, coffee or lemon juice.
2. 110 ml (8 tablespoons) fresh or tinned unsweetened orange juice.
3. 200 ml (1/3 pint) milk.
4. 15 ml (1 tablespoon) concentrated Ribena or rosehip syrup diluted with water.
5. 60 ml (4 tablespoons) Lucozade.
6. 95 ml (6 tablespoons) ordinary Coca Cola.

Special care during pregnancy

The most important action you can take is the careful monitoring of blood sugar. It has been shown that the baby's condition at birth is closely associated with the blood sugar levels of the mother during pregnancy. High blood sugar in early pregnancy is associated with increased malformations in the baby. Excessive tiredness is common in pregnancy and you should be careful of falling asleep and missing meals. This could leave you dangerously hypoglycaemic.

During the last 3 months, women with high blood sugar levels are more likely to have babies that are excessively large. Very large babies cause more delivery problems and are sometimes induced. If this is necessary before 38 weeks the baby is also more likely to have breathing difficulties.

High blood pressure is more often a problem for women with diabetes during pregnancy and so your blood pressure is even more frequently monitored than for other women.

You may also have more regular examinations of your eyes during pregnancy as retinopathy occasionally deteriorates in pregnancy. The availability of laser treatment has meant that much of the anxiety associated with eye troubles has been alleviated.

Will I have to have a Caesarean?

Women with diabetes are more likely to have their babies delivered by Caesarean section because the baby often grows too large for a vaginal delivery. The latest estimates suggest that about 50 per cent of women with diabetes who have babies have them by Caesarean section. Careful blood sugar control throughout pregnancy may help prevent a Caesarean being necessary but you cannot predict this. Most women with diabetes can have a Caesarean section under epidural anaesthetic.

Labour

A diabetic woman's blood sugar has to be extremely well-controlled during labour and so you will be monitored closely and may need glucose and insulin given intravenously. This may mean that your movements are more restricted during labour but otherwise your labour need not be any different to that of a non-diabetic. After the birth insulin requirements will fall back to pre-pregnancy levels, although it may be some time before insulin is required.

Any special problems with the baby?

Babies of diabetic mothers go on producing too much insulin until they are born and then their bodies adjust to their own insulin requirements. While this is happening, they need to be watched to avoid the danger of hypoglycaemia and so may be taken into the Special Care Unit for a while.

Babies born to diabetic mothers often look more 'bloated' due to excess fat. This gradually disappears and the baby will become a normal size after a few months.

Breastfeeding

Can a woman with diabetes breastfeed?

A mother with diabetes can breastfeed successfully if she takes certain precautions in her own eating habits. The important thing is to eat more carbohydrate to replace that being used to feed the baby. You will also need to adjust the times when you eat this extra carbohydrate according to when the baby feeds so as not to become hypoglycaemic. If your blood sugar is low during a feed, the baby is likely to seem less than satisfied at the end of the feed, so you should eat while breastfeeding. If you are still very overweight after the birth, you may not need to take this additional carbohydrate, but seek advice from your diabetes specialist.

Will breastfeeding affect diabetic control?

For most women it will not. For a few women there may be a slight effect such that you need to take less insulin.

Will the baby be adequately nourished?

Yes – all studies have shown that a baby breastfed by a diabetic mother grows as well as that of a non-diabetic mother.

Is there any form of contraception I cannot use?

Because of the increased risk of heart attacks, the combined birth pill is usually not recommended to women with diabetes. However, the new low-dose combined pill carries only a very small risk. The progesterone-only pill is also deemed safe for women with diabetes but is not as effective a form of contraception on its own.

The IUD has also been shown to be less effective in many diabetic women and is associated with an increased incidence of infection, so it should usually be avoided. It seems that the lining of the womb behaves differently in a woman with diabetes, which gives rise to the high failure rate.

Will my child be different?

Women with diabetes, as with other conditions, may be concerned about the effect that their diabetes has on their children's health and performance at school. An interesting study carried out in Belfast compared a group of children of diabetic mothers with another group with non-diabetic mothers. They looked at minor health problems (such as frequent colds, persistent earache, wearing glasses, being overweight, fainting, travel sickness, etc.) and behavioural problems (such as irritability, restlessness, being disobedient). They were also interested in absenteeism from school.

The findings of this survey were encouraging. They showed no difference between the children of diabetic mothers and those of non-diabetic mothers. There were no more health problems, no more behavioural problems, and no more absenteeism from school due to the mother's diabetes.

Diabetes: a case history

Lack of knowledge can increase fear and like most mothers undergoing a first pregnancy, I was apprehensive. My uncertainty was increased by the fact that I was 33 and a diabetic on insulin. Despite being a trained nurse, my knowledge of diabetes and pregnancy was scant and pessimistic. My fears proved unnecessary, however, and I now have a healthy red-haired daughter, 22 months old, and am contemplating the next pregnancy.

I hope the following points arising from my own experiences will be useful to other prospective diabetic mothers.

1. There are risks attached to diabetes and pregnancy, but do not forget that there is some risk in all pregnancies, so do not be discouraged.

2. Pre-conceptual care and a planned pregnancy with good diabetic control and a healthy, high fibre, reduced-fat diet with plenty of fruit and vegetables is advisable for at least 6 months prior to conception. Good liaison with your diabetic care team is necessary here.

3. Early diagnosis of pregnancy is helpful, so try to keep a record of periods after you stop using any contraception.

4. Practise monitoring your blood sugar 4–5 times daily once you have conceived, and make contact with the diabetic care team as soon as possible, maintaining liaison as necessary throughout your pregnancy. Monitoring becomes your security, keeps you out of hospital, helps you know your diabetes, and aids good diabetic control for your and your baby's welfare.

5. Hypoglycaemia in the first few months may be a problem but this passes. I found that my symptoms altered and became less distinct. Hypoglycaemic reactions could make driving dangerous so I stopped driving long distances and always performed a blood glucose test prior to setting out. I also carried glucose sweets everywhere. Some form of identification stating that you are a pregnant diabetic may be a good idea. I believe that the law treats a hypoglycaemic attack while driving similarly to driving under the influence of alcohol or drugs, so be careful.

My husband was away in the early months, so I used friends to check on me each day in case I should have a bad hypo. My colleagues at work were particularly good in this respect. Do not be afraid to ask for this sort of help.

6. In my case considerable increase in the insulin dose was necessary at 28 weeks, which is not unusual as for some reason the pregnancy gives a resistance to insulin at this point. Be advised by the diabetic team. I was using the Novopen with 4–5 injections a day. I felt keeping out of hospital was important.

7. Attend your regular check-ups. I saw the diabetic team every 2 weeks and went to the hospital antenatal clinic at 14, 22, 28 and 32 weeks, and then every 2 weeks until I was induced at 38 weeks. I was given an ultrasound scan every time I attended antenatal clinic to check on the baby's size. It was comforting to see the baby growing well as the ultrasound staff interpreted the image on the scanner. It would have been helpful to have had a combined diabetic and antenatal clinic, but the local situation and positions of the hospitals precluded this, although there was close liaison between the diabetic and obstetric consultants. I also visited my GP for checks in the early weeks but it did mean an awful lot of visits to clinics. A small price to pay for excellent care, though.

8. For me, an induction of labour was not as bad as some people had led me to believe. I opted for an epidural so that I would be awake for a Caesarean if necessary. This again was personal choice. Luckily I had a fairly normal labour with a forceps delivery. My husband did hourly blood sugar checks during labour which was helpful.

9. The epidural was wonderful and allowed me to enjoy labour. I did not feel deprived as I was able to breathe through some contractions prior to this pain relief. It would have been exhausting to carry on for 12 hours, though. You maintain mental control with an epidural too. Labour was a very positive experience.

10. Do not be frightened of the drips and monitors as the midwife will explain things and you can watch your labour progress. Not all consultants believe in induction at 38 weeks but in my case it was thought safer. It is something to be discussed on an individual basis.

11. I was unprepared for a rather bloated baby who had to go to the Special Care Unit due to hypoglycaemia at birth. Apparently babies can become rather large even in fairly well-controlled diabetics and can be at risk from hypoglycaemia. More insulin is produced by the infant inside the mother, which increases the foetal size. Babies of diabetics go on producing too much insulin when born until their little bodies adjust to their own insulin requirement. It does not mean that the baby is diabetic.

The stay in SCU is usually only 12–24 hours until it is certain that the danger of hypoglycaemia has passed. During this time 4-hourly blood glucose monitoring and 4-hourly feeding takes place. Artificial feeds are used until the mother is producing enough milk. One must put the baby to the breast before the artificial feed, or use the breast pump to express milk, in order to encourage one's own milk supplies. Even if your baby is in an incubator longer than 24 hours, breastfeeding is still possible. Do make sure that you state your preferred method of feeding and ask the staff for help.

12. The bloated look soon fades, but baby may lose more weight than usual in hospital due to the loss of the excess fluid that caused the 'diabetic cherub' appearance. My little girl took a month to regain her birth weight, which caused needless worry until it was realised that the birth weight may have been misleading.

13. After the birth I was unable to reduce my insulin to pre-pregnant levels. I believe this is unusual but may have been due to breastfeeding or the altered lifestyle – I had worked physically hard as a nurse until the 28 week point of my pregnancy.

14. Breastfeeding was no problem and is very rewarding, but there is a need to include extra carbohydrate in the diet. It is all too easy for one's own care to be overshadowed by the needs of the baby. I did go hypoglycaemic at first but a change in long-acting insulin overcame this problem. The symptoms of hypoglycaemia have returned although they are still not as pronounced as they were prior to pregnancy.
15. Spacing one's family is advisable so as to allow the diabetes to settle down between pregnancies.

In conclusion: a diabetic pregnancy can be a healthy and happy event. A sensible, positive attitude, close liaison with the medical and obstetric team, the support and help of one's partner, and a little extra care can lead to healthy babies. I can only wish other diabetics a happy parenthood – it is worth the effort.

(Written by and reproduced with the kind permission of Angela Goble.)

Contacts

The British Diabetic Association
10 Queen Anne Street
London W1M 0BD
Tel. 01-323 1531

This is an exceptionally good self-help organisation and provides an excellent range of information for women contemplating pregnancy. Since 1984, it has also been supporting a nationwide network for women with diabetes who want to share the experiences of motherhood with others.

The B. D. A. produces a regular bulletin called *Balance*.

References

British Diabetic Association (1986) *The Diabetes Handbook*, Thorsons.

Burden, A. C. (October 1985) 'Diabetic control during pregnancy', *Practical Diabetes*.

Byrne, E. and Hadden, D. (April 1983) 'Will your child be different?', *Balance*.

Lowy, C. (January 1983) 'Pregnancy and diabetes survey', *Balance*.

*Reyroft Hollingsworth, D. (1984) *Pregnancy, Diabetes and Birth – A Management Guide*, Williams and Williams.

Steel, J. (1987) 'Having a baby', *Balance*.

Steel, J. and Johnstone, F. (1986) 'Prepregnancy management of the diabetic', in Chamberlain, G. and Lumley, J. (eds) *Prepregnancy Care*, John Wiley.

Whichelow, M. and Dodderidge, W. (February 1984) 'Diabetic mothers and breastfeeding', *Balance*.

(* Publications that may prove difficult for readers without a medical education to follow.)

Further reading

Cummins, M. and Norrish, M. (1980) 'Follow-up of children of diabetic mothers', *Archives of Disease in Childhood* 55(4):259–64.

Steel, J. M. (1987) *Coping with Life on Insulin*, Chambers.

There is an excellent chapter on sex and pregnancy.

Knopfler, A. (1989) *Diabetes and Pregnancy*, Optima.

Chapter twelve

Epilepsy

What is epilepsy?

(See Table 12.1)

To have epilepsy is to have a recurrent pattern of fits or seizures. Most people develop it in childhood although there are incidents of epilepsy developing during a first pregnancy. This is believed to be coincidental rather than brought on by the pregnancy.

Who gets it?

One person in 100 has some type of epilepsy – there are many different types of epileptic fits and they can affect people of any age, sex, race or intelligence. It is estimated that 0.5 per cent of women (i.e. 1 in 200) of child-bearing age are affected by a continuing tendency to epileptic seizures.

How is it caused?

Often the cause is not known. For some, the cause may relate to birth difficulties, head injuries, the result of diseases or other medical reasons. In each instance, the disturbance begins in the brain, and because the brain controls all our actions and feelings, the effects may be widespread in the body.

Can it be cured?

No, but in most cases it can be controlled using drugs as prescribed by a doctor.

Table 12.1 Epileptic fits

Type of fit	What it looks like	What can be done by an onlooker
Absence (affects the whole brain)	The person looks blank for a few seconds and then returns to activity.	Very little. Be kind and understanding.
Tonic clonic (affects the whole brain)	The person may cry out and fall. The body jerks and the skin may turn blue. The fit will last a few minutes. The person may be tired and confused afterwards.	Keep calm. Try to protect the head. Let the fit run its course. DO NOT move the person unless they are in any danger. DO NOT put anything between the teeth.
Partial (affects part of the brain)	It is variable. The person may appear confused and repeat movements or smack lips or both, automatically. The fit may be quite long and the person will be confused afterwards.	DO NOT try to stop them. Remove harmful objects and guide them away from danger. Talk quietly.

It is not necessary to call an ambulance or doctor unless the person is injured or does not regain consciousness within a few minutes.

Source: The British Epilepsy Association leaflet on epilepsy.

Can a woman with epilepsy have children?

There is no reason why not, and you are unlikely to be discouraged from having children by your doctor. If possible, you should discuss the matter with your doctor prior to conceiving so that your drug intake can be safely managed.

Will my baby get epilepsy?

Very unlikely. Whether a baby inherits the condition depends on the cause of epilepsy in the mother, and only in a very few women is there any genetic risk of passing the epilepsy on to the child. Discussing the matter with your doctor will help decide whether you should have genetic counselling.

Will it affect fertility?

There is no evidence to suggest that epilepsy impairs fertility. Occasionally women taking anti-convulsant drugs such as Epilim may develop a loss of or change in periods, but this can usually be put right by changing the dosage.

Contraception

Most anti-convulsant drugs interact with the contraceptive pill and women taking these will need a slightly higher dose of the pill. Otherwise there is a danger of unplanned pregnancies so an alternative form of contraception needs to be used as well.

Other forms of contraception are all available to a woman with epilepsy. If a coil is fitted to a woman who has not had children, it may be advisable to have it done under a light anaesthetic to avoid the possibility of the stretching of the cervix causing a reflex faint. This can lead to a convulsant attack.

Drugs and risk to baby before conception

If you have had no seizures for 2 – 3 years you may be advised to have your anti-convulsant treatment gradually withdrawn before any planned pregnancy. Otherwise, ideally, before becoming pregnant, you should be taking a single anti-convulsant which should be enough to control your epilepsy but not so much that side-effects appear. A small amount of folic acid should be taken before you become pregnant. Other vitamins may be necessary and calcium supplements may be a good idea as some anti-convulsant drugs can interfere with the normal production of these.

The risk of anti-convulsant drugs to the baby, if properly managed, is small. At the moment the medical view is that a woman who is at risk of seizures should continue with anti-convulsant medication whilst she is pregnant, if possible with a single drug. If epilepsy is not controlled, there is certainly a high risk to the mother if she develops uncontrolled attacks late in pregnancy, and there may be some risk to the developing baby too if attacks occur frequently.

What is the risk to the baby?

There is a risk that anti-convulsant drugs may cause some kind of abnormality in the developing baby. Some abnormalities caused by drugs in newborn babies are reversible and this slight risk has to be balanced against the risk of uncontrolled attacks in pregnancy. Doctors are still uncertain about how great the risk is, although so far it seems to be small.

It seems that a woman with epilepsy, even if she is not taking anti-convulsant drugs, has a slightly increased risk of producing a 'damaged' child. The normal risk is 2 per cent (i.e. 2 in every 100 children born in this country have some kind of abnormality). The risk for a woman with epilepsy who is not taking anti-convulsant drugs is about 4 per cent. The risk to a woman taking such drugs goes up to 5–6 per cent.

The risk is therefore quite small and most women do find it acceptable, particularly as some of the malformations are correctable once the baby is born. It is important, however, that you obtain professional advice, preferably before conception, so that informed choices can be made.

There is little evidence to suggest that any drug (apart from older anti-convulsant drugs no longer used) carries more risks than any other if given in non-toxic doses. The risk may be slightly increased if two or more anti-convulsant drugs are taken whilst pregnant.

Special care during pregnancy

During pregnancy the blood level of most of the anti-convulsant drugs should be checked fairly often and this check should be continued for 2 – 3 months after the baby is born. With some drugs a slight increase in dose may be necessary towards the end of the pregnancy, followed by a slow reduction once the baby has been born. Vitamin K needs to be given towards the end of the pregnancy and to the baby to prevent bleeding problems associated with some anti-convulsants.

Effect of pregnancy on epilepsy

There is no way of predicting the effect on seizures during a first pregnancy except it seems that those with very frequent seizures are, unfortunately, likely to get worse.

Women with pre-existing epilepsy who have had a prolonged period without seizures are unlikely to get recurrences during pregnancy.

Pregnancy usually has little effect on the frequency of seizures. Not a lot is known about this, but in at least 50 per cent of women there is no change in the attack frequency during pregnancy. In some women, there is an increase which may be due to the effect pregnancy has on blood levels of anti-convulsant drugs, although an increase often occurs in the first 3 months of pregnancy, suggesting that some hormonal or fluid retention factor may cause a reduction of anti-convulsant blood levels. A few fortunate women may experience a complete absence of seizures while pregnant.

By and large, subsequent pregnancies in any one mother follow much the same pattern.

Special note

As a problem quite separate from epilepsy, convulsive seizures due to a complication of pregnancy – eclampsia – may occur in the later stages of pregnancy. In this complication, a sudden marked elevation of blood pressure produces changes in the blood vessels in the brain, resulting in generalised seizures. It is to avoid this that the taking of blood pressure at every antenatal visit is so important and complete bedrest advised if even a moderate elevation is noted. It is not known whether a woman with epilepsy is more likely to get eclampsia during pregnancy.

What pain relief in labour?

Some women with epilepsy find that pethidine used for pain relief in labour may have a convulsant effect. Women who know that they have attacks if they overbreathe should make sure that this information is passed on to their midwife or doctor so that fast, shallow panting, which is commonly used in the later stages of delivery, is avoided.

Can I breastfeed?

Most anti-convulsant drugs get into breast milk to some extent. The benzodiazepines (drugs like Valium) do so to a considerable extent and may produce an unacceptably sleepy baby. Tegretol also gets into breast milk readily, but despite this most women taking Tegretol can breastfeed satisfactorily. None of these drugs is actually harmful to the growing baby. The baby, it should be remembered, will already have been exposed to the drugs in your womb. Again check with your specialist or GP about the drugs you are taking.

Looking after baby

Even a woman having frequent fits can safely rear a child on her own if necessary by taking certain precautions. The obvious ones relate to changing, feeding and bathing the baby. The British Epilepsy Association produces a sheet of practical advice for mothers with epilepsy.

How will my child understand my seizures?

Children do not fear epilepsy unless they are taught to, and a happy family life and normal bonding are completely possible if family and friends support this. Useful children's books explaining epilepsy:

What Difference Does It Make, Danny? by H. Young
The Detective Story by P. Rogan
Learning about Epilepsy by R. Beran

All of the above are available from the BEA.

Epilepsy: a case history

I was 33 when I had my first child. I suffer from temporal lobe epilepsy and before I became pregnant I was having partial fits a few times a month, usually during my sleep. Although having epilepsy is not particularly nice I can live with it, so my concern about having a child who developed epilepsy was not significant as I knew that the risks were small.

My greatest concern was my drug intake. I was taking Epilim and Tegretol and wanted to know whether the drugs would affect the baby if I got pregnant. I found my consultant neurologist tried to be reassuring but seemed rather evasive in his answers.

My pregnancy was a traumatic one – I suffered increased seizures which led to more tiredness and headaches. I also had what I can only describe as 'manic' states due to upsets in brain chemistry as a result of several fits close together. During these states I felt slightly insane: everything became slightly exaggerated visually and my thoughts became strange and terrifying. I was also worried after each fit that my baby might be affected as the full-scale ones were quite violent. My GP was unhelpful and at one point said impatiently, 'Oh, you epileptics are all the same!' I have since changed GP.

I found the NCT classes very helpful and was put in contact with another epileptic mother, which I found very reassuring, particularly the advice she was able to give about child care.

My labour started normally and everyone at the hospital was very helpful. I produced a healthy 8-lb girl and had no fits during labour. My memory of the moment is of feeling extraordinarily emotional and exhausted as if I had just achieved the most enormous feat of my life – like climbing Mount Everest.

I had asked my consultant whether it would be all right to breastfeed and he had checked the drugs I was taking for safety. I breastfed my daughter right from the start and had no problems in hospital. I came home after 7 days, tired and rather nervous of the responsibility of looking after the baby. It took me a few weeks to sort out a routine.

After the baby the nature of my fits changed and I have more during the day and less in my sleep. I felt that this could be related to being more tired and feeling more stressed looking after a child full time. Since going back to work and taking up meditation I have found the epilepsy easier to control.

My daughter is a bright, energetic and beautiful child, which is a great relief to me as I was always concerned that the cocktail of drugs and the seizures would affect her in some way when I was pregnant. She has brought us a great deal of happiness and I look forward to a more relaxed and confident pregnancy next time.

Contacts

The British Epilepsy Association
Anstey House
40 Hanover Square
Leeds LS3 1BE
Tel. 0532 439393

References

Betts, T. A. (1982) 'Women's health and epilepsy', *Epilepsy Now*.

*Dalessio, D. J. (28 February 1985) 'Seizure disorders and pregnancy', *The New England Journal of Medicine*.

* Hopkins, A. (21 February 1987) 'Epilepsy and anti-convulsant drugs', *British Medical Journal*.

(* Publications that may prove difficult for readers without a medical education to follow.)

Further reading

Hopkins, A. (1984) *Epilepsy – The Facts*, Oxford Paperbacks.

Royal College of Midwives (1988) *Guidelines for Mothers with Epilepsy*, Royal College of Midwives.

Chapter thirteen

Hearing impairment

What is a hearing impairment?

A generally accepted definition of deafness includes all people who cannot hear or understand the spoken word with or without a hearing aid. There are many more people with partial hearing loss than people who are completely deaf. People may be born deaf, become deaf in childhood or, most commonly, become hard of hearing in adulthood.

Who gets it?

About 1 in 50 people in the UK have some degree of deafness. It is popularly associated with old age but many younger people suffer from it. There are an estimated 11,000 women of child-bearing age in Britain who suffer some degree of hearing loss.

How does it affect daily life?

One of the major problems facing people with a hearing impairment is that the disability is invisible, so that other people often are not aware of the need to cooperate to aid communication.

The most obvious effect of a hearing impairment is on all spoken communication, whether it is face to face or from the TV and radio. This is very isolating and often means that people with a hearing handicap from an early age have not had as effective an education as they should, so, for example, reading and writing skills may not be as advanced. This usually happens because the hearing loss is not diagnosed until late, not because they are any less intelligent. If the deafness occurred at an early age, speech may be affected too.

Problems of social isolation and lowered self-esteem often arise as a result of the difficulties in communicating – especially since the onus is almost always on the person with a hearing impairment to understand, rather than the hearing person to learn to communicate more effectively.

What is the cause?

There are many forms of hearing loss and they have many causes. In the age group which I am looking at – women in their child-bearing years – the most common type of hearing loss is that due to hereditary otosclerosis. Other less common causes are chronic infection of the middle ear, meningitis in childhood, tumours, accidents, and congenital deafness due to German measles in the pregnant mother.

Can it be cured?

Hereditary otosclerosis can be operated on with great success nowadays, and full hearing restored in most cases. However, the operation is not performed until the hearing loss has deteriorated to a certain level as there is a small risk associated with the operation that the person will be left with a completely dead ear.

Other forms of deafness can sometimes be improved by an operation, but in most cases hearing aids are used to lessen the hearing loss. Hearing aids need to be given together with adequate information about how to get the best out of them. For example, if all a hearing aid does is increase the volume of sounds around you but not the clarity, it is not going to be of much use.

What is the risk that the hearing impairment will be passed on to the child?

Between half and a third of deaf people have inherited their deafness, and there are several forms of deafness that can be passed on. Ask your Ear, Nose and Throat specialist for advice on this if it is a concern.

How will pregnancy affect my hearing condition?

Otosclerosis

It is now recognised that the change in hormone levels during pregnancy can cause further deterioration in hearing, particularly if both ears are affected by the otosclerosis. The deterioration in hearing usually occurs in the later months of a pregnancy and is likely to happen again in subsequent pregnancies.

Ménière's disease

This is very rare, but as it is affected by pregnancy, I will make a few comments on it. The disease affects the level of the fluid in the inner ear and so affects balance. Women with Ménière's suffer attacks of deafness, tinnitus, and acute vertigo when balance seems to go completely. Drugs can help reduce the severity of the attacks but the disease cannot be cured completely.

Hormone changes during pregnancy are thought to lessen the number of attacks although they may reoccur after delivery. In a few cases the Ménière's may actually get worse during pregnancy. The medical management during pregnancy is to avoid the use of drugs completely during the first 12 weeks but to make diuretic drugs available in the second trimester if the attacks become more frequent. A woman with Ménière's needs to be watched even more closely towards the end of her pregnancy for signs of swelling ankles. An attack has no effect on the health of the baby although, obviously, one has to avoid dangerous falls.

Other forms of hearing impairment are mostly unaffected by pregnancy.

What problems may I encounter in pregnancy and labour?

There are few forms of deafness which will physically affect your pregnancy. The problems you are likely to face are purely those of communication and getting adequate and full information.

Ideally you should have an interpreter who is not your partner, so that you are able to get information and make decisions in a 'neutral' space, just like any other woman. It should be a matter of pride for antenatal care providers to take the initiative and seek out interpreters for women with hearing difficulties – after consulting them first. I realise this is not easy, but professionals making contact with local self-help groups may be a first step in locating such interpreters.

The best you can do is to find out as much in advance about what to expect during antenatal examinations, classes, hospital ward, labour room, etc. The booklet produced by the Two-Can Project is highly recommended for this purpose. The other precaution you can take is to make sure a hearing partner, friend or relative accompanies you and keeps you informed as to what is being said.

If you are to have a Caesarean section, your hearing aid will be removed before you go into the operating theatre. Make sure there is someone who knows how to reinsert it afterwards so that you don't miss out on what is going on when you come round. Midwives will not necessarily remember this, so point it out beforehand.

Other possible problems are highlighted in the two personal accounts that now follow. I hope professionals will find them as valuable as mothers-to-be in understanding the sort of worries that exist for women with hearing impairment.

Hearing impairment: case history 1

I am 32, a civil servant, and have a 2-year-old daughter. I am also expecting another child early next year.

My mother first noticed that I had a hearing impairment when I was 2 but I received no help (such as hearing aids) until I was 16. When Anna was born my hearing loss was 60–70 db but it has now deteriorated to 80 db. As I have otosclerosis there is every reason to believe that my hearing will further deteriorate during this pregnancy.

My first pregnancy was unplanned: I had no intention of getting pregnant as the situation in my ears is inoperable, and I had been told that my condition was likely to deteriorate as a result of pregnancy. The registrar at the Ear, Nose and Throat clinic I attended had told me to ask my doctor about having babies when I got married, but I had decided that I did not want to suffer the deterioration. My attitudes on this have changed as I have matured and come to accept my deafness, so I believe I can and will adapt to ongoing and, possibly, progressive deafness.

My experience of babies was fairly limited – I have a sister 10 years younger than me so I remembered her as a baby but that was about it.

I was keen to find out as much as I could about pregnancy and my own condition when I learned that I was pregnant. During the course of doing my own research I discovered that oestrogen is a primary factor in otosclerosis.

At the antenatal clinics I couldn't hear when they called me, so I had to take my mother along as a spare pair of ears. The doctors invariably had foreign accents which I couldn't switch on to. They seemed not to notice that I had asked my notes to be headed 'deaf'.

I attended the antenatal classes run by the midwives locally (again taking my mother as my ears), but I did not find them very useful. The reason for this was they gave us a printed plan of what would be covered in the course of classes but then did not follow it or cover everything. Things like exercises and relaxation were not fully covered nor were things like bottle-feeding.

As I worked for the DHSS at the time, I was able to tap their knowledge at source for some of the information I needed. I worked until 2 weeks before the baby was due.

I went into labour spontaneously and went to hospital about 5 hours before the baby arrived. In general the midwives did not know how to react to deafness – this was probably not helped by the fact that my speech is perfect. They did not realise that if I could not see their lips I could not understand what they were saying. Much of their conversation seemed to be addressed to my bottom or feet! The doctors were the same. They perceived me as a normal hearing person until I explained (to each and every one). Then they got flustered or embarrassed.

My mother attended the labour with me (she had 5 children so she was an old hand) but didn't find the staff very supportive. She was struck by how no one made any effort to see whether I had heard anything or understood what was going on – particularly at times of stress. I don't know how I would have coped without her.

My daughter arrived but had to have her airways cleared out and to be warmed up. After 5 minutes I was able to hold her. My emotions at that time were relief –'I shan't do that again in a hurry' – joy, exhilaration, achievement, wonder – all rolled into one.

I spent 7 days in the hospital in a room on my own as I was testing a new flashing device. Anna had to be taught to suck as she seemed not to be interested at all. As a result I got very swollen and sore breasts. My first day home was a complete disaster. I was on my own, Anna wouldn't stop crying, I burnt the dinner, she wouldn't stop wanting to suck . . .

We had a bumpy first few weeks with Anna vomiting violently and producing vile yellow diarrhoea. The health visitors thought it was because I wasn't feeding her properly but eventually the doctor recognised that she needed specialist medical attention and she now attends Great Ormond St Hospital and is on a very restricted diet. She is thriving at last. I often believe that if it were not for my higher education I would never have got anyone to believe the severity of the situation.

I do have a lot of worries about the future, particularly as I am very isolated from other deaf people. I worry about my need to rely on relatives to escort me to hospitals; my possible future isolation; whether people in groups will take me for an intelligent deaf adult or a moron. As I work full-time I cannot go to playgroups or meet mums, but even so I am frightened when I go to new groups that I won't be able to hear.

Anna is not yet old enough to understand my disability completely but every morning she 'gives me my ears' so that I can talk to her. I try to explain it by putting my hands over her ears to block out the sound and then telling her that Mummy hears like that all the time. But on the whole I believe in not forcing explanations on her unless the situation warrants it or she asks why.

Hearing impairment: case history 2

I am 43 and have a stepson of 11 and an 'own' child of $2^{1}/_{2}$, and we will soon be adopting a deaf child of 4. I am a teacher of the deaf and am married to a hearing person who is head of CE in a deaf school. My hearing loss was caused by meningitis at age 5. I am stone deaf – people say only a few are, well, I am. I have no response to sound.

My only worries prior to getting pregnant were about getting full information and access. I did not seek any specialist advice about my deafness as I knew it would not be passed on to the child. I did seek help getting pregnant. I became pregnant fairly quickly after a hilarious time due to several misunderstandings about, for example, the timing of intercourse to lead to pregnancy.

I had some experience of babies as, being 40, I had many friends with young children. I had a very enjoyable pregnancy with no particular problems except occasionally feeling that I wasn't as fully informed as a hearing mother might have been.

I attended antenatal classes at which my husband interpreted, but I would have appreciated the information being given in the context of deafness. I would have liked to go to exercise and relaxation classes but when there was no interpreter available there was no point going as it turns into a frustrating rather than relaxing experience.

At the hospital antenatal clinics I would tell the Sister I was deaf and where I was sitting waiting so they could fetch me rather than expect me to respond to my name being called out. I would have liked a full-time interpreter separate from my husband, especially on the day of labour when he was trying to cope with giving me emotional support.

When I went into hospital on the day of labour, a midwife asked me if I had been to the toilet and I said yes. When I was on a drip I realised she meant had I emptied my bowels. As it was, it was too late and going to the toilet afterwards to empty my bowels was agony! An example of oral miscommunication.

The baby was 1 week overdue so I was induced and had a very long-drawn-out labour. The midwives were very good and made me feel it was managed the way I wanted. I had an epidural in the end and my daughter was delivered by forceps.

I had to depend on lip-reading and signing which was difficult in a dark room and between labour pains. The midwife was most interested in my deafness and I had to remind her of the reason for my being in the delivery room!

Our daughter was born with club feet but we were able to hold her straight away. We were ecstatic and not at all hung up about her feet. (They were not, of course, related to my having a hearing impairment.) She has since had a couple of operations to straighten them and has had no problems with walking, etc.

In the postnatal period in hospital I had a few problems with breastfeeding, again because of inadequate information, but got there in the end. I also had great pain on walking and then a midwife cut one stitch as it had turned septic. I had thought the pain was normal!

As most communication with staff was verbal, I think there was a tendency to shorten or paraphrase vital information and this gave rise to some of these problems.

Back home my husband was a great support and I was much pampered for a couple of weeks while we got into a routine. I was very conscious of my deafness and kept peeping at the baby to make sure she was still breathing. We had special equipment to alert me to her crying, etc.

Looking back, I'm not sure what I would have done differently – I wanted a more natural birth but lack of full on-the-spot information led me against it. I would also have liked to have met more mothers but I was too wrapped up in looking after the baby and too worn out. I have not joined any mother-and-baby groups as I don't really like baby talk and also felt my deafness would be a barrier.

Our daughter is bilingual (she signs and speaks). Once she signed to everyone but now is more careful whom she signs to. I won't explain my deafness in one way – just say 'I can't hear you' and then gradually build on that.

My only worry about the future is society's attitude to differences which is bound to touch my daughter, but hopefully by that time she will have seen that differences can enrich people's and society's life.

Contacts

The Royal National Institute for the Deaf
105 Gower Street
London WC1E 6AH

British Association for the Hard of Hearing
7/11 Armstrong Road
London W3 7JL

Breakthrough Trust
Deaf-Hearing Integration
Charles W. Gillett Centre
Selly Oaks College
Birmingham B29 6LE

The Ménière's Society
98 Maybury Road
Woking
Surrey GU21 5HX

Can put you in touch with others.

SENSE
Association for Deaf–Blind and Rubella Handicapped
311 Gray's Inn Road
London WC1X 8PT

The following organisation aims to help profoundly deaf adults achieve greater independence and integration by obtaining literacy and information. It produces two excellent booklets: a guide to antenatal clinics (£1) and one to relaxation classes (80p). Both incorporate signs and graphics to aid understanding and are available from:

The Two-Can Project
Rycote Centre for the Deaf
Parker Street
Derby DE1 3HF
Tel. 0332 366083

In Kent, John Brown has set up the Hi centre for deaf/hearing integration. This is to provide information and social contacts for hearing impaired people of all ages:

Hi
MCSC
Marsham Street
Maidstone
Kent ME14 1HH
Tel. 0622 687187

References

*Elbrond, O. and Jensen, K. (1979) 'Otosclerosis and pregnancy', *Clinical Otolaryngology* 4:259–66.

*Gristwood, R. E. and Venables, W. N. (1983) 'Pregnancy and otosclerosis', *Clinical Otolaryngology* 8:205–10.

*Oosterveld, W. J. (1985) *Ménière's Disease – a comprehensive appraisal*, John Wiley.

(* Publications that may prove difficult for readers without a medical education to follow.)

Further reading

For mothers-to-be: the chapter for deaf and partially hearing parents in

Cornwell, M. *Early Years – You and Your Baby*. Available from the Disabled Living Foundation.

The chapter was written with the help of a partially hearing mother and is particularly insightful.

For nurses there is a very comprehensive booklet:

Royal College of Nursing (1985) *Guidelines for Nurses working with the Hearing Impaired in Hospital*, Royal College of Nursing.

For all hospital staff the RNID have produced a leaflet, *The Deaf Person in Hospital*.

For antenatal teachers there is an excellent reference:

Baranowski, Elaine (April 1983) 'Childbirth education classes for expectant deaf parents', *Maternal Child Nursing Journal* 8.

Chapter fourteen

Heart disease

Heart disease covers a wide variety of conditions, a few of which are seriously disabling, although the majority are not. However, since pregnancy places a considerable additional burden on even a healthy heart, it becomes particularly important for women with *any* type of pre-existing heart condition to have expert assessment so that close supervision can be given if necessary during and after pregnancy. This is to minimise the risk to your own health and to ensure a healthy baby.

If the heart disease has not already been diagnosed, pregnancy may be a time when pre-existing problems are brought to light. If there is any history of heart disease in your family, or any recollections of childhood rheumatic fever, any suggestions by you of chest pain or difficulty in breathing, your obstetrician may seek further evaluation of the condition of your heart by a cardiologist.

In such instances, the earlier a heart condition is detected, the more can be done to ensure the safety of both you and your baby. In exceptionally rare cases, it may be necessary to consider termination of pregnancy, if it poses a threat to your own life. Surgical treatment of heart conditions can be performed during pregnancy if absolutely necessary but there is obviously more of a risk involved to both the baby and yourself.

This chapter is concerned with those heart conditions that are most likely to affect a woman in her child-bearing years: congenital heart disease and rheumatic heart disease.

What is heart disease?

Congenital heart disease means that a person has been born with something wrong with the function or formation of the heart which will affect the way it works. There are a great variety of such defects. There may be a narrowing at some point which means that the pumping chamber behind has to work harder to push the blood through; there may be a hole between the two sides of the heart so allowing blood to flow from one side to the other; sometimes the connections to the veins or arteries are faulty, or a part of the heart may be missing. Some of these abnormalities are very slight, some are more serious and require treatment.

Rheumatic heart disease is caused by rheumatic fever, usually in childhood, and causes damage to one or more of the heart valves. Surgery is usually eventually required to replace the damaged valve.

What causes heart disease?

The cause is not always clear. It is estimated that 90 per cent of congenital heart defects result from a combination of genetic and environmental factors (such as drug intake, infection, or exposure to radiation); 8 per cent are caused solely by an identifiable genetic defect, and the last 2 per cent are attributed to solely environmental factors.

Rheumatic heart disease results from an infection entering the blood (following a sore throat, for example), spreading to the joints, and accumulating in the heart valves. It results in scarring of the valves which, over the passage of time, develop calcium deposits, which interfere with their function.

How many people are affected?

Congenital heart disease

About 8 babies in every 1000 are born with an abnormality of the heart. Modern diagnostic and treatment methods mean that a vast majority of these now grow up to lead ordinary healthy lives.

Published reports of studies in Europe, North America and Australia suggest that congenital heart disease occurs in about 1 in 100 pregnancies.

Rheumatic heart disease

In developed countries like Britain new cases of rheumatic heart disease are becoming rare and it is less common than congenital heart disease.

However, there are still many cases to be found amongst women of child-bearing age who contracted the disease in their own childhood years. On the whole, the severity of the disease when it does occur is less nowadays because of the availability of better treatment.

How does it affect daily life?

Again, this depends on the particular condition, its severity, and how it is being treated. In severe cases it can be extremely disabling as all activity and physical exertion is restricted. However, many people with heart conditions are able to lead full and active lives by use of appropriate drugs and/or as a result of surgery.

Can a woman with heart disease have children?

In the vast majority of cases, if the heart condition has been treated (for example, by surgery), or is under control through drug treatment, a woman with heart disease can have children safely. Most women with congenital heart defects have uneventful pregnancies and women with rheumatic heart disease that has been treated are also likely to be able to have children safely.

There is evidence to suggest that having children will not affect the longer-term survival of a woman with either congenital or rheumatic heart disease.

There are a few heart conditions that may make pregnancy inadvisable. These include raised blood pressure in the lungs (pulmonary hypertension), a condition known as Eisenmenger's Syndrome, and a postnatal disorder affecting heart tissue (puerperal cardiomyopathy). If you have any of these conditions your cardiologist may suggest sterilisation, as pregnancy could threaten your life.

However, if you decide to go against this advice and become pregnant, it is most important to see an obstetrician and cardiologist early in pregnancy. You may again be advised to have a termination but this will not be forced on you, and with such severe heart disease, it would be absolutely essential to have expert advice and care throughout the pregnancy.

Another condition, known as Marfan's Syndrome, was also once thought to fall into this category but recent evidence suggests that it is not as dangerous as previously thought and, except in the severest cases, a safe pregnancy is possible if closely supervised.

What is the risk to the baby?

There are three different risks to consider. The first is whether the baby is more likely to have heart disease if one or both parents have it. Genetic counselling should be sought from your cardiologist or a genetic counsellor.

It is estimated that if neither parent has heart disease the probability that their first child will have heart disease is less than 1 in 100. Congenital heart disease in either parent increases this risk.

There is also some evidence of a genetic predisposition to rheumatic fever, in other words, a child may be more likely to be vulnerable to rheumatic fever if either of his parents or any of their close family has been affected by it. There seems to be no evidence, however, to suggest that if a parent has suffered rheumatic fever the child will be born with any congenital heart defects.

If your heart abnormality is congenital, there is thought to be an increased risk that the child will have a similar form of congenital abnormality, but this risk varies with different types of heart defect. It also seems that if the mother has a congenital heart condition, the child is more at risk than if the father has such a condition. If both parents have congenital conditions the risk is greater than if only one is affected.

Your cardiologist or genetic counsellor will look closely at the incidence of heart conditions (not just in you and your husband but also in close relatives) before explaining what risk there may be to your child. Most serious cases of congenital heart disease in the baby can now be diagnosed in the first half of pregnancy by ultrasound tests. This enables you to consider abortion if the condition is one that is not amenable to surgery in infancy and you are therefore not prepared to go ahead with it.

The second area of risk to consider is how your heart condition will affect the growth and development of the baby. In general terms, the greater the reduction in your heart's function the more concern there will be for your baby's normal growth and development. Research suggests that women with cyanosis (a blueness arising from shortage of oxygen in the blood that is caused by some heart and lung conditions) are likely to have babies who are very small at birth. However, obstructions in the mother's heart, or leaky heart valves that impair its output, are less likely to affect the baby's growth during pregnancy.

The third risk to consider is that due to any drugs or treatment you might need to be taking to ensure your own health through and beyond

144

pregnancy. Your cardiologist and obstetrician should collaborate to ensure that the risks are minimised. In general, most drugs used to treat heart disease are safe, but drugs may be changed during pregnancy, so it is important to tell your cardiologist of your intention to become pregnant.

Other precautions to minimise the risk of the child being born with a heart defect apply to *all* pregnant women and include avoiding all infection by getting immunised well before pregnancy and avoiding excessive X-rays. Also, remember that the older you are the greater the risk of having a child with Down's Syndrome; over half such children have congenital defects of the heart.

Pre-pregnancy preparation

It is very important to seek medical advice *before* becoming pregnant so that any risks are minimised before you embark on the pregnancy, and any surgical treatment or adjustment to your drug consumption can be carried out.

A cardiologist will discuss the issue of pregnancy and childbirth with any young woman he treats – if possible, long before she chooses to start a family. The discussion and consideration at this early stage is important as it may affect the nature of the treatment she receives. For example, a young woman requiring a valve replacement would be better given an animal graft rather than a mechanical valve since the former is less likely to require anti-clotting medication and will therefore pose less of a risk to a foetus.

Since infection of any sort is potentially more dangerous to a pregnant woman with heart disease, you will be helped to prevent it through immunisation. Immunisation against polio, rubella, influenza, mumps, measles, and tetanus should be carried out well before the commencement of a pregnancy (at least 3 months).

Family planning

It is important to plan each pregnancy so as to be in the best of health yourself and to minimise the risk to the baby. Intervals of at least one or two years between pregnancies are usually advisable for this reason.

Contraception methods should be discussed with your cardiologist. Oral contraceptives may pose special hazards to women with heart conditions and need to be prescribed with care. The oestrogen component of the Pill is suspected of being dangerous to women with heart disease but such women may safely use low oestrogen or progesterone-only pills. Women over 35 and/or women who smoke should not use oral contraceptives.

The use of the IUD is also potentially dangerous to women with heart disease because of the risk of infection and is therefore not usually encouraged. If for any reason, an IUD is used, it is important to use one of the smaller ones and to ensure sterility at insertion. Preventative use of antibiotics is recommended. There should be regular examination after insertion and you should report any increases in vaginal discharge, cramping, backache or prolonged bleeding.

Barrier methods such as diaphragms and condoms are effective if used properly and can provide women with heart disease the safest form of contraception, particularly between pregnancies.

Will heart disease affect fertility?

There is no evidence to suggest this. There is a very slight possibility that if you have a congenital heart condition there may also be a congenital abnormality of your reproductive system, so gynaecological investigation may be suggested by your cardiologist before you embark on motherhood.

Will a Caesarean be necessary?

In the majority of cases a normal vaginal delivery will be possible, but you may be discouraged from a 'trial of labour' (for example, to see whether you can push the baby out if it is in a breech position), as the strain on your heart may pose a threat to your own life.

The obstetrician, cardiologist, and anaesthetist will have to compare the relative risk to your heart of the burden of a vaginal delivery that may go on for a prolonged period of time, with the disturbance to your heart associated with anaesthesia and surgery over the short and predictable period of time of a Caesarean delivery. The decision will be made on the basis of their understanding of your heart condition as well as your obstetric condition.

Special care during pregnancy

During a normal pregnancy your body undergoes an almost miraculous number of adjustments to cope with the developing baby. In particular, there is a significant increase in the amount of blood circulating in your body so as to feed the placenta and thus support the growing foetus. This increased volume of blood places additional demands on the heart and circulatory system – the rate at which the heart beats and the amount of work it has to do increases, and there are corresponding changes in the resistance put up by the blood vessels, so that they enlarge and blood pressure decreases.

Since no aspect of the body works in isolation it follows that there will be a number of other changes that will take place as a result of, or, as well as, the circulatory changes. For example, kidney function is also affected. These changes in the internal workings of the body may give rise to a variety of symptoms such as light-headedness, fatigue, swelling of the fingers and ankles, prominent veins, heart murmurs, and so on – even in women with a normal heart.

The changes of pregnancy are tolerated well by most women, but if there is some pre-existing weakness in the functioning of the heart, it may not be able to cope with the additional demands. That is why it is so crucial to seek medical advice before becoming pregnant and why you will be very closely monitored during your pregnancy with checks perhaps as frequent as once a week. If there are any signs that your heart is not coping, the cardiologist will be able to advise on changes in your drug treatment or, in severe cases, even surgery.

The medical management you receive during your pregnancy will include close watch on the composition of your blood (to check for signs of anaemia, for example) and urine, and your blood pressure; the rate at which your heart beats will be controlled and any arrhythmia will be suppressed by use of drugs.

If you have an artificial heart valve, the anti-blood clotting drugs such as warfarin that you have been taking before pregnancy, have a small but definite risk of causing skeletal and brain damage to the baby. Unfortunately there is no completely safe alternative. Some doctors have tried administering heparin injections early in pregnancy but these are not as effective in preventing blood clots forming. These are very dangerous to the mother in about 1 in 4 pregnancies. However, at the end of pregnancy, warfarin cannot be used because of the bleeding risk in the baby. Therefore women who are taking warfarin for heart disease in pregnancy are often asked to come into hospital early so that they can have heparin by drip infusion for about two weeks before the baby is born.

147

Infections often increase the symptoms of heart disease and so it is important to avoid them as far as possible and to treat them early if they do occur. If you have a history of rheumatic fever, antibiotics may be prescribed to prevent recurrent infections and consequent rheumatic fever.

Iron deficiency anaemia is a common effect of pregnancy and usually poses no danger to a pregnant woman, but if your heart condition is such that you embark on pregnancy with lowered haemoglobin and iron stores, the anaemia could put an extra burden on the heart and bring about heart failure. Therefore close monitoring of your blood before and throughout the pregnancy will enable identification and prevention of dangerous anaemia.

Excessive weight gain during pregnancy is also to be avoided since this can make breathing difficult and place an additional burden on the heart. For a woman of normal build, a weight gain of about 25 pounds is recommended. You may also be asked to weigh yourself daily so as to detect signs of fluid retention which in a woman with chronic heart disease may indicate developing heart failure.

Hypertensive heart disease is unusual in pregnant women but pregnancy-induced hypertension (high blood pressure) is not, and needs to be closely watched in all cases but particularly in women with heart disease.

Normal obstetric procedures will be taken to monitor the progress of your baby with the likely addition of more ultrasound checks to check for normal development and growth as these may be impaired if the function of your own heart is severely compromised.

You will probably be discouraged from doing any antenatal exercises which could strain your heart, but it is worth talking to an obstetric physiotherapist about your posture and ways of doing everyday things such as getting out of bed in such a way as to minimise exertion.

Tiredness is also likely to be more of a problem and you will be advised to take as much rest as possible, not just at night.

Heart surgery during pregnancy

This is very unlikely to be necessary for the vast majority of women with heart disease in pregnancy. However, there are several important heart complications that occur with increased frequency during pregnancy in women with heart disease and your obstetrician, GP, and cardiologist will be watching out for these throughout. Heart failure can occur for a number of different reasons and can be fatal, so it requires prompt recognition and treatment. If it occurs, drugs will be administered to control it and you will be admitted to the intensive care unit as soon as possible to establish the cause and to prevent any further damage. In the rare cases where heart failure cannot be controlled with drugs, surgery may be needed.

Operations on heart valves such as mitral valve surgery and heart valve replacement surgery have now been performed frequently on pregnant women with considerable success, but in general they will only be carried out if there is an imminent danger to the mother's health. However, closed mitral valvotomy which does not need bypass is so safe in pregnancy that it may be recommended when women are well because it is known that the condition deteriorates as pregnancy continues.

The timing of any surgery in pregnancy is important. It is thought that the best time to perform surgery is between 12 and 20 weeks, as it is during this period that the risk to both mother and foetus is lowest.

In all heart operations in pregnancy, the heart rate of the foetus will be monitored continuously throughout the operation: although it has been shown that it will drop while the mother's heart has been stopped, it usually regains its pre-operation rate within 90 minutes or so of the operation. The chances of delivering a healthy baby at full term after heart surgery seem extremely good.

Surgery to correct congenital heart defects should take place many years before the age of child-bearing and should not be necessary during pregnancy. There are occasional reports of such operations during pregnancy, and the majority of these have been successful.

Labour

If a normal vaginal delivery is anticipated, you will be watched very closely throughout labour to ensure that your heart is coping. This will involve connecting you to various monitors and so may restrict your movements. The second stage may be shortened by use of forceps so as to deliver the baby more quickly and thus limit the strain of pushing.

Many obstetricians and cardiologists will prescribe antibiotics during and after delivery to prevent infections in all women with structural heart defects.

Pain relief

The range of pain relief that you will be offered will be the same as for any other woman. For many women with heart disease epidural anaesthesia is particularly advantageous because it reduces the work done by the heart in labour. There are a few conditions, such as Eisenmenger's Syndrome, where epidural anaesthesia may not be considered safe, but these are rare.

Postnatal care

For most women with serious heart disease, the dangers associated with pregnancy do not end with delivery. Continued preventative measures against infections are necessary by use of antibiotics. You will also be encouraged to get up and walk about as soon after delivery as possible (you may be given elastic support stockings to wear for this) so as to avoid dangerous blood clots.

Your baby will be examined closely for any signs of heart defects. If you have been on anti-coagulants just before delivery, your baby may be given vitamin K at birth to counteract their possible effects on the baby's own stores of this vitamin.

Breastfeeding

If you have been in good health while pregnant and your heart has been able to cope with the strain of pregnancy, it should certainly be able to cope with breastfeeding.

As has already been mentioned, there is a rise in the total blood volume through pregnancy, and this includes a progressive rise in blood flow to the breasts which peaks during the first month after delivery in women who breastfeed their babies. For a few women with a serious heart condition this increase in blood flow could put too much of a strain on the heart and so breastfeeding may be discouraged. The risk of mastitis (infection due to blockage in the breast milk ducts) is an additional hazard to women with serious heart disease.

Each woman's condition will obviously require individual assessment but if breastfeeding is important to you, you should make this clear to the obstetrician caring for you. In the few exceptional cases where it is decided that breastfeeding will be too dangerous, steps will be taken to suppress lactation in the early days and to prevent breast engorgement. This may be done by use of drugs or by tight binding of the breast, use of ice-packs, and painkillers.

Contacts

British Heart Foundation
102 Gloucester Place
London W1H 4DH

The Chest, Heart and Stroke Association
Tavistock House North
Tavistock Square
London WC1

The above are national headquarters but both organisations have regional centres and the BHF also has local groups actively raising money for research. They both provide factsheets on general aspects of heart disease but, at the time of writing, neither has any specific information relating to pregnancy.

The CHSA sees itself as providing support and has established a contacts register called INTERHEART which aims to put people in touch with others in their own area who have had similar heart conditions.

INTERHEART co-ordinator:
Mike Preston
Tel. Leicester (0533) 431194

Marfan Association
70 Greenways
Courtmoor
Fleet
Hants GU13 9XD
Tel. 0252 617320

Disseminates information about the Marfan Syndrome and can put you in touch with other women.

References

*Metcalf, J., MacAnulty, J. H., and Veland, K. (1986) *Burwell and Metcalf's Heart Disease and Pregnancy* (2nd edn), Little, Brown and Co.

This extremely comprehensive American book covers all aspects of diagnosis and management of heart disease in pregnancy. It is also a very good source of relevant references on the subject.

*De Swiet, M. (1989) 'Heart disease in pregnancy', in De Swiet, M. *Medical Disorders in Obstetric Practice*, Blackwell Scientific Publications.

*Szekely, P. and Snaith, L. (1974) *Heart Disease and Pregnancy*, Edinburgh: Churchill and Livingstone.

Jukes, K. (June 1988) 'Breastfeeding under threat – a case study of a mother with a heart condition', *NCT New Generation* 7(2):34.

(* Publications that may prove difficult for readers without a medical education to follow.)

Chapter fifteen

Multiple sclerosis

What is multiple sclerosis?

Multiple sclerosis (MS) is a disease of the nervous system which is characterised by periods when the symptoms get worse (relapses) combined with periods when they get better or even disappear (remissions). In some people the disease is of a progressive nature which results eventually in mild or severe disability, but this is not always the case.

In MS, the myelin sheath, a protective coating around the nerves in the brain and spine, breaks down in many places and so affects the transmission of messages from the brain to the rest of the body. This gives rise to symptoms such as pins and needles, loss of coordination, slurred speech, and difficulty in regulating the strength and size of movements including walking.

Loss of vision in one eye for a few weeks is often the first sign of the disease, but this is only temporary. A few people with MS also suffer epileptic fits.

Who gets it ?

MS is a predominantly North European and North American disease. It affects women more than men. In Britain, 1 in 1000 of the population is estimated to have MS. The figures for women with the disease are 1.7/1000 in the 25 – 35 age group and 2.4/1000 in the 35 – 45 age group. These are approximately double the rates for the disease in men. It should be remembered that these figures cover the whole range of MS sufferers, from those who have a very mild form to those with a severe disability.

How does it affect daily life?

Every person with MS is affected differently, even if she has had the disease for the same length of time as someone else. However, for the benefit of those not familiar with the condition, the following list gives the major ways in which it may affect daily life:

- Holding things is difficult.
- Walking becomes progressively more difficult.
- Bladder and bowel control is often impaired.
- Muscle spasms in legs may cause problems during some activities such as walking or sex.
- Emotional ups-and-downs associated with the uncertain progress of the disease are common.
- Extreme fatigue is often a debilitating aspect.

What is the cause?

Much research is being carried out, but as yet the causes are unknown.

Can it be cured?

As yet, there is no proven cure for MS. Various treatments are given to try to reduce the symptoms but there is no evidence that any of them stops or reverses the course of the disease. Some doctors prescribe short courses of steroids if the MS has deteriorated recently, as these may help the person recover more quickly, but there is no conclusive evidence that they make a major difference in the long run. A variety of other treatments (evening primrose oil, hyperbaric oxygen) have also been suggested, but the evidence for their effectiveness is similarly lacking.

Is it wise for a woman with MS to have children?

Years ago, women with MS were told that they should not have children because it would make their condition worse, but this is not the view of most neurologists nowadays and they will now not dissuade a couple from having children if they so wish.

The question that most women with MS want answered is whether or not having children will affect the progress of their MS, but there is no conclusive evidence to answer this either way. The medical trials required are highly impractical to carry out. You need to find women of comparable age and at the same stage of the disease and then observe the course of the disease in the group that have children and compare it to a group that don't – AND you have to take into account other factors that might affect the MS in individuals. Not easy. Attempts have been made to do such research, but different conclusions have been reached and in many cases the size of the sample groups has been too small to be significant.

The main considerations will therefore be practical, not medical. Looking after children is hard work and only you will know how you will cope. It is often advised that women with MS should only have one or two children, but again, this is for practical reasons. Some experts usually also advise waiting for a period of time after a relapse before becoming pregnant. This is not unreasonable as it makes sense to be stable before embarking on something so major as a pregnancy. On the other hand, if it seems that the MS is progressing rapidly, then it may be better to have the baby as soon as possible, before the condition becomes too advanced.

So should you have children? The decision is yours. One neurologist I spoke to put it like this: 'Yes, MS does make people's lives unpredictable but we all have to face that – anyone could get run over tomorrow; one in three of us is likely to get cancer, etc. The uncertainty of the disease should be kept in context. If a couple really want children then they should go ahead.'

Will MS affect fertility?

There is no evidence that MS affects fertility in a woman.

Drugs and risk to baby

Most drugs should be stopped before you conceive. These include drugs you may be taking to stop painful spasms; control of urinary frequency or incontinence; and any long-term therapies such as Imuran, cyclosporin or hyperbaric oxygen. You are unlikely to have a relapse during pregnancy (see page 157), so steroids such as ACTH are not likely to be necessary. Doctors would not knowingly prescribe steroids during pregnancy, but even if you did become pregnant while taking them, it is very unlikely that the baby would be affected.

New drugs are coming into use all the time and your neurologist will call the Drugs Advisory Office to check on the up-to-date information about the use of any particular drug in pregnancy.

Will the MS be passed on to the baby?

As with arthritis, it is not uncommon for MS to affect more than one member of the same family, but this does not mean that the disease is inherited. There is no evidence to suggest that you will pass the disease on to your baby and therefore this should not be a major consideration in whether or not to go ahead and have children.

Will the MS harm the baby?

There is no evidence to suggest that a child born to a woman with MS is any more likely to be damaged.

How will the pregnancy affect the MS?

There is usually an improvement of the symptoms during pregnancy and relapses are rare during the pregnancy, especially after the first trimester. However, as every sufferer knows, the course of MS in any one person is unpredictable, and this remains so during pregnancy.

Relapses after childbirth are common. Various studies have shown that relapses are likely to occur within the first year after the birth (usually 3 – 6 months after) and that the majority of women recover fully.

Research into the overall effects of pregnancy on the progress of the disease suggests that there are none. If a relapse occurs it is now thought that childbirth has merely delayed or brought forward a relapse that would have occurred anyway.

In practical terms, a growing baby will press on the bladder, perhaps making bladder control even more of a problem. Your balance may also be affected as your centre of gravity changes.

Will a Caesarean be necessary?

If your MS is such that you may have difficulty in pushing the baby out, you are slightly more likely to have a Caesarean. Otherwise you are no more likely to have one than any other woman.

Special care during pregnancy

Try to stay active but avoid getting over-tired. If you are able to do any of the antenatal exercises, do so, paying special attention to pelvic floor exercises. Since fatigue is likely to be a problem for many women with MS, energetic exercising is to be avoided. However, gentle toning exercises, preferably supervised by your neurological physiotherapist, should be possible in order to tone abdominal and pelvic floor muscles and maintain good circulation.

Pain relief during labour

You will be offered the same range of pain relief as any other woman in labour, with the possible exception of epidural anaesthesia. This is because anaesthetists may be wary of relapses – including heaviness in legs – in MS patients following childbirth: these may be blamed on the epidural, even though it is unlikely to be the cause. Discuss the policy in your hospital beforehand.

Labour

Depending on how severe the MS is, your ability to push may be affected and you may need the help of forceps to get the baby out. Otherwise your labour is as unpredictable as any other mother's.

Breastfeeding

There is no reason why you should not breastfeed. If you start taking any drugs again, check with your neurologist as to their effects on a breastfed baby.

Contraception

The Pill has been linked with having a negative effect on MS sufferers so should be avoided.

Multiple sclerosis: case history 1

At the age of 26 I had what seemed like a stroke and my eyes were temporarily blinded as if by bright sunshine. I recovered but was then diagnosed as having MS.

It was obviously a shock. I was newly married and my first question was, 'What about children?' Both the neurologist and my GP were very reassuring and told me to go ahead and lead a normal life. I was told that pregnancy might either help or make my symptoms worse, but that they could not predict which it would be.

Dave and I decided to go ahead and start a family straight away. I conceived immediately and had a good pregnancy. At the time I was not disabled and so it was difficult to tell whether the pregnancy had any good effect on the MS. My job as a speech therapist at a child development centre meant that I was fairly well informed about children and I did read quite a lot of general stuff about pregnancy. There was nothing on pregnancy and MS and I was discouraged by my GP from joining the MS society or talking to anyone else with MS. In retrospect I regret this as I think it might have helped me to cope with a lot of the uncertainty.

I was induced at my own request as I was 10 days overdue and very uncomfortable. I had a good labour and went home with my son Peter much like any other new mother. During Peter's first year I had two bad attacks and over the next couple of years my condition did deteriorate.

By the time I became pregnant for the second time I was disabled: I was walking with a stick, my coordination was very bad, and I had a definite tremor in my left hand. It was a big decision to go for another child, but we decided to go ahead before my condition made it impossible.

I had far more problems in my second pregnancy, particularly with back-ache and excessive tiredness. I don't think there was any particular improvement of the MS either. I also went to a different hospital because we had moved, and the midwives really didn't seem to know what MS was or how to handle me.

The labour second time round was not so good – I didn't feel as well prepared and became very emotional. I needed a lot more in the way of drugs. I panicked in the postnatal ward because it was crowded and my eyes couldn't handle the excessive stimuli. I wish I could have had a separate room but there were none available at the time.

Coming home with Haley was a real shock. It suddenly hit me that I couldn't do a whole lot of things with her that I had done with Peter – just ordinary things like carrying and changing her had become awkward and dangerous because of the MS. I coped with the help of family, friends and a home-help, though I found it very difficult to accept help, particularly in the early days. I wanted to show that I could manage and I was fighting to be normal.

Peter is now 5 and Haley 2¹/₂ and both are a real delight. I think Peter is much more sensitive because of my disability and clearly understands quite a bit. For example, I once asked him to throw me a ball and he immediately said, 'You can't catch the ball 'cos you can't move quick enough.'

I can't. And I can't play football with him either. I tire more and more easily and seem to have become very emotional – I cry and giggle a lot. Dave has been very understanding but he also cries sometimes when he sees other women with more advanced MS and sees how I might become.

Most of the time we are very positive about it all and make sure the children don't lose out. I have been in touch with a few other mothers with MS whose support we have both benefited from. I hope I will not have put you off if you have MS and are reading this to help you decide whether to have children. I really do feel it has been worth it and it has brought a great deal of happiness despite the hardship.

Multiple sclerosis: case history 2

I am 26 and have three children aged 4, 3, and 1. My MS was diagnosed 6 years ago and I immediately rushed out and bought Judy Graham's book on the condition and read it from cover to cover. I was determined right from the start to be positive about it and to try to lead as normal a life as possible. To begin with this was not too difficult as the symptoms were fairly mild – fatigue and occasional clumsiness.

I had read somewhere that MS can harm fertility, so I was a bit worried, but in fact I conceived fairly easily. When I first became pregnant I went to my GP and he advised me to have an abortion because he didn't think women with MS should have children as it would make their health worse in the long run. I explained that we were prepared to take the risk and from then on he was cool but not unhelpful.

The pregnancy was a worrying one as I suffered bleeding on and off throughout. The doctors seemed unsympathetic and kept threatening a Caesarean.

I didn't attend any classes and was given no special advice about diet or exercise. At the time I didn't know whom to ask. The obstetrician said I should be induced, so I was. The labour was long and I was given an epidural early on because of the MS. The baby was born bruised and couldn't breastfeed which I was disappointed about.

I didn't have a relapse until the baby was 2¹/₂ months old and it lasted until he was 6 months. My husband was extremely unsympathetic and became quite violent. I also discovered I was pregnant again. The second pregnancy was tough because I had the baby to look after. However, the MS definitely improved after the early months. At about 33 weeks I became unable to walk because the baby was pressing against my sciatic nerve, so was forced into a wheelchair.

There was some difficulty in ascertaining the date my baby was due and my daughter was induced at 35 weeks. Again, the labour was long and the second stage was particularly tough as I couldn't push very well. My daughter was whisked away without my being able to hold her.

I was in a wheelchair on the postnatal ward and was ignored by the other mothers except, surprisingly, for one who was blind. We seemed to have a lot more in common and got on very well. I came home after 4 days and my mother was at home to help.

My MS is not as bad as some people's. I have a heaviness in my legs which makes walking difficult but still possible, and I don't suffer too much from shakiness. With a bit of help I can manage fairly well and I don't think the children have suffered because of my illness.

My advice to other women with MS contemplating pregnancy is that you should stick to your instincts and ignore other people. You know what you can cope with best.

Multiple sclerosis: case history 3

My first pregnancy took place before my MS was diagnosed (following a bout of back trouble) and it was a very healthy and happy pregnancy and short, well-managed labour. My second pregnancy couldn't have been more different.

We had tried to get information from my GP and neurologist about the risks involved: my GP had told us there was a finite risk of problems and, when pressed, my neurologist said he wouldn't recommend having 10 children. This sounded to us like a signal that we could go ahead, which we did, particularly for James's sake – we wanted him to have a brother or sister.

I had a particularly bad miscarriage which drained me both physically and emotionally, but we decided to try again. This time the pregnancy was really bad all round. I was violently sick, constantly tired, and had great problems with walking and balance. My GP was very supportive throughout which helped a great deal.

The MS did not improve at all during the pregnancy and in fact the symptoms got a lot worse. Steroid levels are supposed to go up during pregnancy, so you should feel better. I can only assume that I was unlucky enough to have an atypical reaction.

I had been told by the obstetrician that I would have to be induced as it was unlikely that I would go into labour normally, and lack of sensation would make feeling the baby move impossible. He wanted to avoid the stress effects of a labour and to get things over quickly.

I was seen by the obstetrician once a fortnight from about 4 months into the pregnancy. From 1 month before Tom was born I started getting very strong contractions – they were certainly a lot stronger than any Braxton-Hicks contractions I ever had, so much so that I couldn't walk when they happened. One night I went to hospital believing labour had started, but after 5 hours it stopped, much to my surprise and that of the midwife.

A day before my due date, I got the most appalling headache. I couldn't move my head, which felt as if it would explode. I rang the antenatal clinic and they told me to come straight down. Once there they found my blood pressure was up from its normal 90/50 to 120/80. They felt this was sufficient reason to take me in. (To be fair, the obstetrician had been trying to get me to come in for about 3 weeks, but I didn't want to leave James. He felt I needed to rest but I felt unable to rest with James at home.)

I stayed on the A/N ward at the hospital and was monitored. The obstetrician was away and they could not make any decisions until his return. He came back a week later – so I was 41/40 weeks. He felt that letting the pregnancy go any longer would create too much stress, though hospital policy was no intervention before 42 weeks.

He was willing to try an induction, but with my history of the past month he didn't feel it would be successful. He planned that he should start a drip the following morning and so he would be on hand. If no baby appeared by midday, he would do a Caesarean himself, so he planned to be there throughout.

Unfortunately Tom had other ideas and made his own appearance early the following morning, before the consultant arrived. I was then left alone with Tom for 2 hours with no balance on a high delivery table, even though I didn't need stitches.

After a while they came to move me to a first stage room to await transfer to a local maternity home. I protested, saying the obstetrician wanted me to stay at the hospital. I was told that I had had a normal delivery and that all mothers who had normal deliveries went to the maternity home. I should have made more fuss but postnatal mothers aren't terribly hardy.

The ambulance arrived (3 hours after the delivery). I was told to carry Tom, despite the fact I could hardly stand up myself. On transfer I was in quite a state, suffering from vertigo and absolutely exhausted. At this point my legs decided to join the rest of my body and refused to move properly.

The maternity home was only for non-problem mothers and so I rather non-plussed them. I was told that I would be seen by a doctor the following day and if we were both all right we could go home. I said the obstetrician had told me I would be on bedrest for 12 days but they said that as the birth had been normal this was not necessary. I just wanted to get home and back to my GP. The following day we were declared fit and well despite the fact that Tom had screamed from the moment he was born and that I could no longer stand upright without help.

Once home, I couldn't carry Tom up and down stairs at all and pushed him round indoors in a pram to get from room to room. It was an awful time and I am glad it is over. I can't help feeling that if I had had a Caesarean with the obstetrician around I might well be better now.

The difficulties I encounter bringing up my sons are many. There is the constant tiredness. I am unable to do the things that other mums do like going for a walk to the park or swings. I cannot run after the child if he runs away. If he falls I cannot get to him quickly, etc., etc.

The boys cope well although Tom is too young to understand. James mentions it but accepts it. They know mummy gets tired. The funniest thing was explaining neurology to a group of 3-year-olds at Tom's nursery school. They love the stick I now use and feel they have to look after me. Tom has learnt that if he knocks me from behind I almost always fall over so he sometimes does it if I have told him off.

However tired I feel, I try to help at their schools. Because the other children know me, I am not 'strange'. I think this stops them teasing the boys. Once you understand something it stops being frightening.

Overall I feel that the second pregnancy has proved too costly in terms of what it has done to my family, but no one could have predicted it would turn out this way so I do not regret my decision to have a second child.

My advice is that if a child is important to you then it could be worth the risk – only you can decide.

Contacts

The MS Society
Head Office
25 Effie Road
London SW6
Tel. 071-736 6267

Runs a link service to put sufferers in touch with others in the same area.

ARMS
Action for Research into Multiple Sclerosis
Head Office
4a Chapel Road
Stansted
Essex CM24 8AG
Counselling tel. nos:
071-222 3123 (London)
041 637 2262 (Glasgow)
021 476 4229 (Birmingham)

This self-help group has been a source of great help in education and counselling people with MS and keeps up to date with new research in all aspects of MS.

Some neurologists are sceptical about the way ARMS present this research, suggesting that they often give undue significance to forms of treatment that have not been proved by medical trials, so giving false hopes to sufferers. On the other hand, they accept that ARMS may be pushing them to test treatments that they otherwise would not have bothered with and so one day they might find something genuinely useful. They point out that people often look for new treatments when they are at their worst and find that they get better – but they would have got better anyway, so what significance has the treatment?

References

Forti, A. and Segal, J. (1986) *MS and Pregnancy*. Available from ARMS.

Matthews, W. B. (ed.) (1985) *Macalpine's Multiple Sclerosis*, Churchill Livingstone.

Sibley, W. (ed.) (1988) *Therapeutic Claims in the Treatment of MS*, Macmillan.

Further reading

Graham, J. (1987) *Multiple Sclerosis*, Thorsons.

Barrett, M. (1977) *Sexuality and Multiple Sclerosis*. Available from The Association for the Sexual Problems of the Disabled (SPOD).

Burnfield, A. (1985) *Multiple Sclerosis – a personal exploration*, Souvenir Press.
Has a section on sex, pregnancy, and children.

More difficult to get hold of but interesting reading:

Gilbert, A. E. (1973) *You Can Do It from a Wheelchair*, New Rochelle, NY: Arlington House Publishers.

This is by a mother of four who describes her own techniques for childcare while coping with MS. She stresses the importance of strategic planning and family support.

Belohorec, A. (1985) 'How do you mother when you are disabled?', *The Canadian Nurse* 81:32–5.

A mother of three recounts her thoughts about her ability to carry out a mothering role as she adjusts to her MS.

Smith, A. M. and Meyers, A. B. (1984) 'Family planning and motherhood: experiences of women with multiple sclerosis', *Rehabilitation Counselor Education Program*, Milwaukee, Wis.: University of Wisconsin.

Audiovisual material

Isobel's Baby. Forty-minute video that follows the experience of one woman who has MS, through her pregnancy and first months of motherhood. Available from Arrowhead Productions, 51 Thames Village, London W4 3UF.

Chapter sixteen

Scoliosis

What is scoliosis?

Scoliosis is a sideways buckling of the spine towards a C- or an S-shape. It is a spinal deformity caused during childhood or adolescence and affects no other part of the body or mind. It is rarely disabling nowadays but may cause concern, so I include this chapter for reassurance.

What causes it?

The shape of our backs is partly inherited, partly affected by growth. The shape of our spine changes most rapidly through childhood and adolescence until spinal growth stops at around the age of 25. Children normally have some degree of round back which flattens out during late childhood and early adolescence, but shifting of the delicate balance of weight on the growing spine during this process occasionally throws the flat spine out of alignment, starting the scoliosis. If this happens in girls during early puberty, the deformity is greater because girls grow faster than boys at this time, so the spine is deformed as it grows. At this stage boys have not reached their peak adolescent growth speed, so will be more mildly, if at all, affected.

Obviously what I have described above is a weakness of the spinal column which buckles due to unstable rotational forces during the growth period. Certain medical conditions can make the individual more vulnerable to scoliosis by either weakening the bone material, or adding to the likelihood of rotational imbalance.

Who gets it?

It is estimated that 1 in 10 people have a mild scoliosis but about 1 in 100 have it to a marked degree. Women and men are equally likely to

Figure 16.1

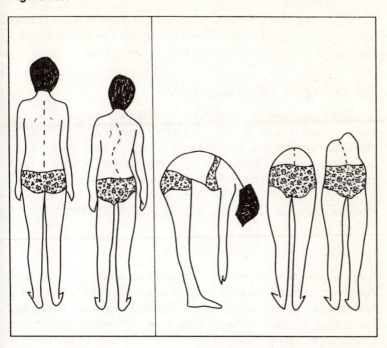

| In scoliosis the spine becomes curved. | Scoliosis can often be detected in a young person by examination of the back while bending at the waist. |

Source: *What is Scoliosis?*, British Scoliosis Association (1987).

get it but the progress of the disease is worse in women, so that ten times as many women as men have severe scoliosis. The reason for this is that growth in puberty is faster in girls than in boys so the curvature becomes more pronounced.

Can it be cured?

Surgery is used to lessen the degree of deformity.

Can a woman with scoliosis have children?

Yes – scoliosis is a benign condition which has no effect on a woman's ability to have or bring up children.

Will the child get scoliosis?

There is a tendency for scoliosis to occur in families, so if one or more relatives has it, a child is more likely to get it. But the risks are still very small and should not affect your decision to have a baby.

Will the pregnancy affect the scoliosis?

No. In the past there was thought to be a link between pregnancy and further deformity of the spine but this is now thought to be coincidental. The spine does not stop growing until the age of about 25 and since many women with scoliosis are likely to have children before this age it may seem as if the further deformity is due to pregnancy, but in fact it would have happened any way. There is not thought to be a hormonal component to scoliosis such that pregnancy itself will affect it.

Special care during pregnancy?

None in particular. A woman with scoliosis should take the same interest in antenatal exercise, a good diet, and so on as any other mother-to-be. It used to be thought that scoliosis could affect lung function but this has now been shown to be very unlikely unless there was severe curvature before the age of 4 or 5. So only a tiny number of women will experience any breathing difficulties due to the scoliosis.

Special care during labour?

Scoliosis has no effect on the shape of the pelvis, so a Caesarean is no more likely to be necessary. The only possible problem that might arise is if epidural anaesthesia is required for pain relief – if the curve is low down it may be difficult to insert the needle. However, in such a case a caudal epidural technique can usually be employed further down your back.

Conclusion

Scoliosis alone does not pose any specific problems to a woman contemplating pregnancy and I hope the above information provides reassurance.

Contacts

British Scoliosis Association
380 Harrow Road
London W9
Tel. 071-289 5652

This also has local groups that work on raising understanding of what scoliosis is.

References

Betz, R. R., Bunnell, W. P., Lambrecht-Miller, E., and MacEwen, G. D. (January 1987) 'Scoliosis and pregnancy', *The Journal of Bone and Joint Surgery*.

* Dickson, R. A. (21 May 1988) 'The aetiology of spinal deformities', *Lancet*.

* Leatherman, K. D. and Dixon, R. A. (1988) *The Management of Spinal Deformities*, Wright.

(* Publications that may prove difficult for readers without a medical education to follow.)

Chapter seventeen

Spina bifida

Spina bifida is a fault in the spinal column in which one or more of the vertebrae (the bones which form the backbone) fail to form properly, leaving a gap or a split. This happens between the 14th and 25th day of pregnancy, so that when the baby is born, the damage is already done. Most people think of spina bifida as a disability that means the person affected will be in a wheelchair. The reality is that there are different kinds and degrees of spina bifida ranging in its effects from the very mild to the very severe.

Spina bifida cystica

This is the most serious form of spina bifida. The visible signs on a baby are a sac or cyst rather like a large blister on the back covered by a thin layer of skin. There are two forms:

Myelomeningocele

This is the most common of the cystica type of spina bifida. Depending on where on the backbone the split occurs, it can cause the most problems. The sac or cyst not only contains tissue and cerebrospinal fluid (the fluid that bathes and protects the brain and spinal cord) but also nerves and part of the spinal cord. The spinal cord is damaged or not properly developed so there is a degree of paralysis and loss of sensation below the damaged vertebrae. The extent of the disability depends on where on the spine the lesion occurs and the amount of nerve damage involved. Most people with this condition experience problems with bladder and bowel control. The majority of babies born with spina bifida

Figure 17.1 Types of spina bifida

	Spinal cord (close up)	Location of spina bifida
	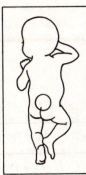	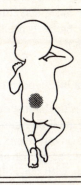

Occulta
Outer part of vertebrae not completely joined. Spinal cord and covering (meninges) undamaged. Hair often at site of defect.

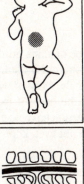
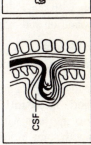

Meningocele
Outer part of vertebrae split. Spinal cord normal. Meninges damaged and pushed out through opening.

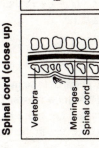
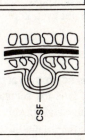

Myelomeningocele
Outer part of vertebrae split. Spinal cord and meninges damaged and pushed out through opening. Possible hydrocephalus.

Source: Spina Bifida and You – A Guide for Young People, ASBAH.

also have hydrocephalus which may leave residual perceptual and learning problems.

Meningocele

In this less common form the sac contains meninges – tissues which cover the spinal cord – and cerebrospinal fluid, but the extent of nerve involvement is usually small and therefore there is often little disability present.

Spina bifida occulta

This is the least serious type of spina bifida. The split in the vertebrae is very small and there is usually no damage to the spinal cord and no nerve involvement. Often the only external sign of its presence is a dimple or tuft of hair on the base of the spine. The vast majority of people with spina bifida occulta have no problems whatsoever related to the condition and often do not even know they have it.

What is the cause and who gets it?

The cause of spina bifida is not known at present. There does seem to be a genetic factor involved. It is the second most common reason for a baby being born with a physical disability and there are more babies born with spina bifida in Great Britain than anywhere else in the world. Within Britain, areas with a high Celtic population such as South Wales and Cornwall have a higher incidence than others. A shortage of, or impaired absorption of, folic acid has also been linked with spina bifida.

The general level of births of spina bifida babies is going down. This is at least partly due to the availability of ultrasound and amniocentesis as antenatal screening devices and abortion being offered if spina bifida is detected.

There are estimated to be about 3 in 2000 babies born with spina bifida in the UK each year. Better surgical and medical treatment during childhood means that more people born with this condition are surviving to adolescence and adulthood now. This means that more women with spina bifida can now contemplate motherhood.

Can it be cured?

Not entirely but, depending on the severity of the initial damage, the baby is operated on immediately and then again throughout childhood to minimise the paralysing effects. At any given time, 10,000 – 15,000 children will be undergoing treatment in the UK.

How does it affect the daily life of a woman?

This depends on severity. In the most severe cases, the entire lower body is paralysed, the person is incontinent and the growth of the lower body is retarded. Usually it is less severe: the paralysis is only partial and there is still some sensation. Bowel and bladder functions can be controlled with assistance if necessary. There may be a partial or total loss of sensation around the vagina but this does not mean that sex is not pleasurable.

Can a woman with spina bifida have children?

Again this depends on the severity of the spina bifida effects. If you have severe incontinence and/or poor kidney function you may be advised against pregnancy as it may pose a threat to your own health. It is possible for most women with spina bifida to have children.

Will it affect fertility?

There is no evidence to suggest this in the case of women. Men with spina bifida may be unable to ejaculate fully, so their ability to biologically father their own children may be more limited.

Will a Caesarean be necessary?

The majority of women with spina bifida have a deformity of the pelvis which makes a safe vaginal delivery difficult or impossible. It may be that your spinal deformity is not so severe and the obstetrician will allow you to try to have a vaginal delivery. However, if it is decided that the best approach would be a Caesarean section, the obstetrician and mid-wives should ensure you are comfortably positioned on the operating table. This is particularly important if you are unable to lie flat on your back as you will need to be cushioned appropriately so as not to cause discomfort after the anaesthesia has worn off.

What is the risk that the baby will inherit spina bifida?

If you have spina bifida or there is spina bifida in your family, then there is a higher risk that your baby will have spina bifida. The risk to the population as a whole is 1 in 500. The risk where one parent has spina bifida rises to 1 in 25 and if both parents have spina bifida, then the risk to the baby is estimated to be 1 in 10.

It is important to see a genetic counsellor who will discuss the risk with you and advise on the use of vitamin supplementation as a way of reducing the risk. You will probably be offered an amniocentesis test (see Chapter 2) once you are pregnant, although a detailed ultrasound scan at 18 weeks' gestation should detect any abnormal development of the baby's spine. If antenatal screening does detect spina bifida, you will be given the option of terminating your pregnancy.

How will the pregnancy affect the disability?

There should be no permanent effect but a few temporary ones, in particular an increased incidence of urinary tract infection and a greater difficulty in transferring and moving around as your centre of gravity shifts with your growing size.

Special care during pregnancy?

You may be advised to take a course of vitamin supplements as these are thought to reduce the risks to your baby of getting spina bifida.

Other problems such as muscle spasms, pressure sores, and kidney care are very similar to those encountered by a woman with a spinal injury (see page 182). Your doctor and physiotherapist should be able to offer you additional advice about dealing with these.

Delivery

If the growing uterus is causing you excessive discomfort, you may be called into hospital for a Caesarean section a few weeks before the 40 weeks of pregnancy are up. If you are to attempt a vaginal delivery, your abdominal muscles should allow you to bear down when the time comes to push. A supportive midwife and careful positioning with foam wedges can help considerably.

Breastfeeding

There is no medical reason why the spina bifida should affect your ability to breastfeed but sometimes positioning the baby comfortably may prove difficult.

Contraception

Talk to your GP about which of the different methods are safe and comfortable for you to use.

Spina bifida: case history 1

I live in Chelmsford and was 26 when my husband and I decided to start a family. I knew other mothers with spina bifida so felt well-informed about how I would cope myself and did not seek medical help until I was already pregnant. I use a wheelchair but am active and was in full-time employment as a legal secretary at the time.

As soon as my GP confirmed the pregnancy he set up a meeting with the consultant obstetrician at the local hospital. There I was interviewed by one of the doctors on the consultant's team. One of the first things he did was to arrange for an ultrasound scan which showed that everything was progressing normally. As a result of this scan I was advised against having an amniocentesis as there is a small risk associated with the test.

It was decided early on that I would have to have a Caesarean section as my pelvis was not suitable for a vaginal delivery. I was given combined folic acid and iron tablets and told to try to stay active. I was monitored closely throughout the pregnancy but had no problems except with my bladder and this was not treated until after the baby was born, so I did not take any medication at all.

I was given a separate room to myself so felt protected from any awkward moments with other mothers (in particular, being stared at).

Although I had intended to breastfeed I found I was too weak after the operation so opted for bottle-feeding.

I felt well-treated by the staff. They did not seem to have any particular knowledge of my disability but on the whole were prepared to listen and offer help when asked. The only exception to this was when, a week after Sarah was born, I developed a severe back-ache; I put it down to a kidney infection and told the nurses. But the doctors insisted on doing a number of tests before coming to the same conclusion a couple of days later. If only doctors listened to the patients when they believe they know what causes their discomfort, a lot of problems might be alleviated.

I came home and was called on by the midwife for 3 weeks. I had no extra help, apart from my husband, and managed well with the baby-care. In retrospect, I feel I didn't have any special problems apart from the ones that all new mothers face with a new baby. As a wheelchair user, my house was already adapted for my needs, and my father had made a purpose-built cot for the baby. I had also attached a velcro strap to the baby changing mat to stop her rolling off it. Since Sarah was about 6 months I have had a home-help for a few hours each week which I find very useful.

My only slight frustration is the isolation that looking after a baby imposes. However, this is now less than when Sarah was very small as I belong to a mother-and-toddler group that meets in a local church hall and also to the local NCT group. I am learning to drive and waiting to pass my test so I can be less dependent on others for transport. My health visitor has been very supportive and a very useful link with the outside world.

We would like to have one more child but are planning to wait until Sarah is 6 or 7 and able to take care of herself. On the whole I feel my experience of childbirth was a positive one and would do nothing different next time around.

Spina bifida: case history 2

I am 31 years old and have two sons aged 6 and 2. I have spina bifida and have been profoundly deaf since 1973. Both my husband and I use wheelchairs.

Before becoming pregnant for the first time, I worried about losing mobility and how I would keep well during pregnancy. There was also a nagging doubt as to whether the baby would be all right.

We saw a consultant and he said there was no reason why we should have a handicapped baby. He advised me to take a course of multi-vitamins for 3 months and I was offered regular scans and an alpha-feta protein test. We didn't seek genetic counselling as we felt happy with the advice we had received from our consultant. I also knew several other women with spina bifida with children who were not handicapped, so this increased my confidence.

I read whatever I could find on pregnancy as soon as I became pregnant myself. I found the books on disability rather negative about parenthood but enjoyed reading general books on pregnancy such as Miriam Stoppard's Pregnancy and Birth Book.

I have communication difficulties with my GP, so any worries I had I tended to share with the doctor in the antenatal clinic at the hospital. There were no access problems but I did find transferring on to a bed more and more difficult as I got heavier and by the end of the pregnancy had to come into hospital on a stretcher.

After a fairly healthy pregnancy, I was admitted to hospital at 29 weeks with high blood pressure but it returned to normal after 2 hours. It was thought to be due to exertion after I had lifted myself on to the ultrasound scan couch. From then on I was always lifted on to the couch. The only other minor problem I had was that my legs swelled dramatically.

I never attended any antenatal teaching classes as, by the time they started, I was too big to travel to them in my car. Nor did I receive any useful advice about diet, exercise, relaxation techniques or what to buy for the baby. In retrospect I regret this but I managed all right.

Four weeks before the baby was born I went into hospital so they could keep an eye on me. I did want to have my baby naturally but the hospital said that they had only ever had one other woman with spina bifida and she had needed a Caesarean. However, they let me try on the understanding that I would have a Caesarean if I got into difficulties.

It was stressed throughout the pregnancy that it was my body and my baby and that they would only intervene if either of our lives was at risk. All the staff were very good and helpful. My husband attended the birth and we were delighted that I was able to deliver our son normally.

I was unable to have a bath during labour because the sides of the bath were too high. Most of my labour was spent upright on the bed and that is how I delivered my son. I held him straight away and felt enormously maternal; tremendously relieved that the baby showed no signs of physical disability and generally happy and proud that I had such a lovely baby. My whole life seemed to fall into perspective.

I went home after 10 days. Learning to handle the baby was not really a problem as I had thought ahead and talked to other mothers with spina bifida and also obtained equipment adapted to my needs from the Social Services. This included a hospital cot specially adapted for a mother in a wheelchair which I was allowed to take home and found very useful. They also adapted a bedside changing table but this was not so good.

REMAP built me a pram frame to attach to the wheelchair – a brilliant idea but unfortunately it doesn't work. I have also adapted a moses basket stand to take a changing mat.

My second pregnancy was more complicated as it was discovered at 29 weeks that I had an excess of rhesus negative antibodies (unrelated to the spina bifida) and would have to have a Caesarean which I did at 39 weeks. I requested it to be done under epidural rather than general anaesthetic but as the anaesthetist hadn't done this before on a woman with spina bifida, we agreed to go for the safe option.

My son was given to my husband to hold straight away but had to be whisked off to intensive care for 4 days. The baby was severely jaundiced because of the rhesus disease: he had to have his blood changed and had all sorts of wires and tapes attached to him everywhere. We were encouraged to stroke him on the first day but I was apprehensive of all the equipment. On the next day I was able to hold him and from then on I was quite happy about handling him.

I have been pleasantly surprised by how easy it has been to look after my children despite warnings to the contrary, though I realise that this is probably because both of them slept through the night from the first day home so I do not get too tired.

We have had no extra help looking after the children although we do have extremely good neighbours who, when they have time, take the children to the shops with them or to play with their own children. This allows me to get on with other things.

My advice to other women with spina bifida who are concerned about having children is to think ahead about how you will look after the child and what equipment and help you might need. For example, we have a local company which does cleaning and I can use it if I am ill or if the children are ill and need more care than usual.

Take stock of your environment and try to find a home where you won't always be worrying about your child running on the road – preferably within reach of toddler playgroups, etc. It's so much easier if you can get to these places yourself. If you can't drive, look and see if there is any such scheme as Dial-a-ride in your area. We have a Homestart organisation in our area and I can ask a volunteer to do something with the children that I cannot manage, such as going to the beach, as there is no way we could have managed with wheelchairs on the sand.

Contacts

Association for Spina Bifida and Hydrocephalus
ASBAH House
42 Park Road
Peterborough PE1 2UQ
Tel. 0733 555488

References and further reading

Drakes, O. (1984) 'Spina bifida and motherhood', *Special Education: Forward Trends* 11(1).

ASBAH *Sex for Young People with Spina Bifida.*

Chapter eighteen

Spinal cord injury

What is spinal cord injury?

The spinal cord is the bundle of nerves running from the base of the skull down the centre of the spine, hidden and protected by the vertebrae (bones) in the back. These nerves carry messages from the brain to the rest of the body so if they are damaged through a spinal injury, partial or complete paralysis of the body is likely to occur.

The site of the damage along the spine determines how much of the body is affected so doctors describe spinal cord injury in terms of which vertebra it is nearest to. There are seven neck (cervical) vertebrae, twelve chest (thoracic) vertebrae and five lower back (lumbar) vertebrae. A T6 injury, for example, is an injury of the spinal cord near the sixth thoracic vertebra and is associated with paralysis of the lower limbs, whereas a C7 injury near the bottom-most neck vertebra could also involve the upper limbs.

Paraplegia is a partial or complete paralysis below the waist. Tetraplegia (Quadriplegia) is a partial or complete paralysis from the neck down.

What is the cause?

Varied, but mostly through road accidents and falls and sometimes through surgery, for example, for removal of tumour. Injury can obviously happen at any age.

How many women are affected?

Accurate figures are hard to come by as records are not adequately kept but it is estimated that in Britain at present about 1000 women of child-bearing age have spinal injuries.

How does it affect daily life?

Mobility and use of legs is restricted, so a wheelchair is needed. Bowel and bladder functions are affected, so management of these becomes a major consideration. Sexual function tends to be less affected in women than in men.

Can it be cured?

As yet, there is no known way of curing spinal damage.

Can a woman with a spinal injury have children?

In the majority of cases, yes. The knowledge that there have been hundreds of paraplegic and quadriplegic women continuing pregnancies to term and delivering normal, healthy infants should provide encouragement to spinal-cord-injured women contemplating pregnancy. Many spinal units recommend that you should wait for 2 years after your spinal injury before becoming pregnant. This is to allow your body to recover as well as to give you time to come to terms with your injury before embarking on parenthood. Many units offer pre-pregnancy counselling too.

Contraception

The combined Pill is not recommended because of the risk of blood clots causing a stroke. Other forms of contraceptive are entirely a matter of personal preference and comfort.

Will it affect fertility?

No – if you were fertile before the injury then you will be again when your periods return.

Drugs and risk to baby before conception

Anti-spasmodic drugs and urinary tract infection control drugs should be reduced or stopped. Your specialist will advise you on this.

Will the pregnancy further harm the woman with spinal injury?

The physical changes of pregnancy greatly increase the normal disabilities of a spinal-cord-injured woman, but if these are anticipated and properly managed there should not be any lasting ill effects after the baby is born.

Special care during pregnancy

As mentioned above, the usual problems of being spinal-cord-injured are accentuated during pregnancy and have to be dealt with appropriately. If you have decided to stop taking anti-spasmodic drugs, it becomes even more important to maintain stretching exercises daily.

Urinary tract infection: the incidence of this increases greatly with pregnancy and you will be advised to take a course of antibiotics each time this occurs. You may also be prescribed a drug to prevent infections.

Pressure sores and deep vein thrombosis: the increased weight acquired during pregnancy combined with the circulatory changes that occur means that the risk of both these increases, and additional measures need to be taken. These include physiotherapy and range of motion exercises – discuss with your physiotherapist. You should take extra care in transferring, as the growing baby will change your centre of gravity.

Will I have to have a Caesarean?

Unless there is an obstetric problem unrelated to your spinal cord injury, there is no reason why you should not deliver the baby vaginally. Research has shown that most spinal cord women can deliver normal babies vaginally.

How will I know I'm in labour?

You are likely to be admitted to hospital in advance of your due date and monitored very closely in the last few weeks of your pregnancy, so it is very unlikely that you will go into labour without knowing.

You will also be told the signs to look out for, such as the stomach going rigid regularly for 30 seconds every few minutes. Even if you can't feel this you will be able to see the abdomen going rigid like a board. Also look out for mucus plug, bloody show and leakage of amniotic fluid.

How will I know when to push if I can't feel anything?

The body goes into labour to produce a baby and the contractions of the uterus will usually push the baby out, with or without your help. In the case of high lesions some assistance may be necessary, for example, vacuum extraction or forceps. There are also often troublesome spasms or cramps of the pelvic muscles which may mean assistance is necessary. In the case of low lesions, you can help by filling your lungs, bearing down, and also applying pressure to the top of your uterus with your hands. A sympathetic midwife should be able to help you with this.

Will it hurt?

If the lesion is complete then you are unlikely to feel any contractions below your waist and so pain relief will be unnecessary. If the paralysis is only partial, you may feel some discomfort and you will be offered the same range of pain relief as any other woman in labour, with the possible exception of epidural anaesthesia.

If your lesion is T6 or above, you are likely to suffer a painful headache with each contraction as your blood pressure soars. This is an unfortunate symptom of autonomic hyperreflexia which is discussed below.

Precautions during labour

The potential problems are:

> early labour
> hyperreflexia
> urinary tract infection
> pressure sores

Early labour

This is common in spinal-cord-injured women, so your obstetrician will probably advise weekly checks after 30 weeks. If dilatation of the cervix is noticed, bedrest in hospital will be advised and a drug will be administered to stop early labour.

Hyperreflexia

If the level of paralysis is T6 or above, there is a high probability that autonomic hyperreflexia may occur during contractions in labour. This is marked by a rapid soaring in blood pressure, headache, blurred vision, nasal congestion, nausea, and sweating below the level of the spinal cord injury.

It occurs in response to pelvic stimulation such as bowel or bladder distension, sexual intercourse, or labour and delivery. The most effective treatment is to remove the stimulus – emptying the bowel or bladder, interrupting sexual intercourse, or delivering the baby as quickly as possible by use of forceps if necessary, or even by Caesarean section. If you have had hyperreflexia before, tell the doctors caring for you so that they can be extra vigilant during labour.

Induction can actually cause hyperreflexia, so it is not performed for women with T6 or above paralysis unless the doctor and delivery room staff are confident in monitoring and managing hyperreflexia.

In Britain, management of hyperreflexia during labour' has been limited to sitting the woman upright at the height of each contraction so the blood pressure drops slightly – enough to prevent a stroke and to take the edge off the pain. In the USA in recent years the use of epidural anaesthesia has been used successfully to treat hyperreflexia during labour. The epidural catheter is inserted at the start of labour but not injected until autonomic hyperreflexia is encountered. Dramatic relief of the symptoms usually occurs within minutes of injection. Epidural anaesthesia blocks the stimuli causing the hyperreflexia and has the advantage that it avoids the possibility of severe hypotension which can occur with the use of anti-hypertensive drugs and prevent exposure of the foetus to such medications. This technique is being introduced in Britain now.

Urinary tract infection

This is unfortunately extremely common despite even the most careful bladder management. Continuous bladder drainage during labour will be maintained so as to avoid the need for frequent catheterisation and a source of autonomic hyperreflexia.

Pressure sores

These are a frequent problem and the midwives should take special care to turn and pad you. This is especially important during a long labour. Leg stirrups could also cause problems and should be used with care.

If stitches are necessary they should be done with care so as to avoid bruising. An episiotomy may be preferable to a bad tear as it is easier to stitch up neatly. Doctors or midwives should not assume that, because you cannot feel any sensation in the perineal area, any less care is required.

Breastfeeding

Women with a spinal cord injury lactate normally and in most cases can breastfeed successfully. The factors to consider are the comfort with which you are able to do so and whether the drugs you are taking affect the breastmilk to a dangerous degree. In purely practical terms, it is far easier to breastfeed than to have to fuss around with sterilising units, bottles, etc.

Postnatal care

Many maternity units that cater for spinal-injured women are still not perfectly adapted in terms of comfortable beds, wheelchair accessibility, etc. You should take extra care in transferring as your newly reduced size will take a few days to get used to and you may find yourself falling around a lot more.

Spinal cord injury: a case history

This American case report is reprinted here as the detail it includes makes it particularly interesting reading.

Jean X, age 30, had sustained a C7 injury and was left paralysed from the armpits down with some weakness in the muscles of her arms and hands. She did not realise she was pregnant for 3 months as she had been taking birth control pills at the time of conception, and the doctor who examined her when she complained of nausea, fatigue, and weight gain told her: 'You're simply gaining weight – what do you expect now that you sit in a wheelchair all day?' Jean's sister insisted that the doctor order a pregnancy test. The result was positive.

Learning that she was pregnant, Jean had doubts about giving birth and raising another child. She was separated from her husband and also now from the partner who was the father of the baby she was carrying. But she had a supportive family nearby and a mother who was keen to help her with her 10-year-old son.

Jean was put in touch with a nurse and childbirth teacher with some knowledge of spinal-injured women. Over the next few months, she and Jean were able to discuss the normal aspects of pregnancy as well as the ones of special concern to spinal-cord-injured women. Because of her injury and advancing pregnancy, Jean was vulnerable to urinary tract infections, skin breakdown, and circulatory problems. She also risked physical injury since transferring in and out of her wheelchair would become more awkward as her uterus grew larger. To prevent these problems, the teacher emphasised the importance of several things – good nutrition, ample fluid intake, meticulous catheter technique, range of motion exercises, skin care, and transfer safety.

They also discussed labour and delivery. Since she would probably not feel her labour contractions, Jean had to be alert for other signs of impending labour. She was told about watching for the mucus plug, bloody show, and leakage of amniotic fluid from the vagina. The teacher also described how the uterus contracted during labour, making the abdomen hard and board-like. At rhythmical intervals, Jean could expect her abdomen to tighten for 30–60 seconds, gradually soften, and then tighten again several minutes later. When she compared these with the Braxton-Hicks contractions that she had already been getting during late pregnancy, Jean remarked that these contractions created pressure and a feeling of not being able to get her breath.

The teacher showed her some breathing techniques to help her relax and cope with this pressure. She also showed her how she could help with the delivery of the baby by filling her lungs and bearing down and applying pressure to the top of her uterus. They talked about hospital procedures, induction, the fetal monitor, the use of forceps, and the possibility of autonomic hyperreflexia occurring during labour. Finally, they talked about postnatal care, with emphasis on the prevention of urinary tract infections, thrombophlebitis, pneumonia, and skin breakdown.

Jean's doctors were concerned that she might not know when labour had begun and suggested she should either come into hospital for the last 8 weeks or be examined closely as an outpatient and induced into labour as soon as her cervix was ripe and slightly dilated. Jean opted for the latter to avoid prolonged separation from her son.

One week prior to her due date she was admitted, ready to be induced. Her time in hospital was 'quite an experience'. No one realised she was paralysed. A midwife, assuming she was in a wheelchair because she was pregnant, asked why she hadn't gotten into bed. A nurse told her to hop up on to the bathroom scales so she could be weighed. When Jean failed to do so she whispered to Jean's sister, 'Why can't she get up?' After learning that Jean was paralysed, the instructor finally turned to her and said, 'Well, you'd never know to look at you.'

Even when the nurses realised that Jean was paralysed, they were still not prepared to handle her special needs. They put her in a bed with a manual crank at the foot, rather than in one with electric controls at the sides. They had never heard of a shower bench. And they put away Jean's sliding board, not realising that she used it for transferring back and forth from wheelchair to bed. Jean reported that the nurses gathered in disbelief when she performed her own catheterisation: 'They couldn't understand how I could do it so easily without even looking when they had so much trouble passing their own patients.'

The day after admission, Jean was transferred to the labour ward and given intravenous fluids to which Pitocin, a contraction-inducing drug, was added. She was 2 cm dilated and her blood pressure was 80/40. Uterine contractions began appearing on the monitor, but Jean had no sensation of them. The labour nurse, forgetting this, repeatedly asked if she was having any.

To avoid decubitus ulcers, Jean was repositioned every 30 minutes. Once, however, she was found to have her toes caught under the bar at the foot of the bed and had to be lifted up towards the headboard.

At 1 pm, 2 hours after the induction of labour had been begun, Jean was still only 2 cm dilated, so her waters were broken and an internal fetal monitor applied to the baby's scalp. Shortly afterwards, Jean began experiencing upward pressure with her contractions that she described as 'a feeling in my throat like the baby is coming up'. Her breathing and relaxation techniques helped minimise this discomfort.

By 1.20 pm Jean's contractions were 3 minutes apart and lasting 70–80 seconds. Her blood pressure was beginning to rise. Because of her Nothing By Mouth status, Jean had missed three doses of Lioresal, a muscle anti-spasmodic. She began having muscle spasms and developed a severe headache.

By 4 pm, Jean had progressed to 5 cm but her headache was excruciating. She needed constant support to help her breathing and relaxation. By this time, Jean's blood pressure had risen to 154/84 – a considerable increase over the 80/40 admission reading. She was given Demerol (pethidine) and Largon (an anti-vomiting drug) intravenously. Her headache subsided and her blood pressure, after peaking at 160/90, decreased to 124/70.

Finally, at 4.55 pm – 5 hours after labour had begun – Jean was fully dilated and ready for delivery. In the delivery room, the doctor decided to use a birthing chair to maximise the assistance of gravity. With six people lifting her in a sheet, Jean was moved to the birthing chair and safely positioned. She was told to start pushing whenever she felt the pressure of a contraction in her throat and neck. When a contraction came Jean filled her lungs, pulled up with her arms, and pushed as hard as she could. At the same time, the nurse applied constant fundal pressure to Jean's uterus. Within 2 to 3 pushes, the baby's head crowned.

Suddenly Jean's headache returned and her blood pressure soared to 160/90. The doctor quickly applied low forceps and delivered a healthy 6lb 9oz boy. Within 5 minutes Jean's blood pressure returned to 120/70.

The baby had been safely delivered, but the lower portion of Jean's uterus had clamped down, trapping the placenta inside. With difficulty, the physician began removing the placenta. Like a see-saw, Jean's blood pressure rose again and her headache returned. Once the placenta was out, her blood pressure quickly dropped.

Jean spent the rest of the night carefully observed by the nurses in the labour ward. The next morning she was transferred to a room near the nurses' station on the postpartum floor. While the staff were attentive and helpful, Jean still felt she was something of an attraction during her postpartum stay. Otherwise, she was much like the other new mothers on the floor. Babycare classes were held in Jean's room for her convenience. She decided not to breastfeed or have rooming-in, but the baby was brought to her for all scheduled feedings. Unfortunately, Jean developed a postpartum urinary tract infection despite rigorous preventative measures. To treat the infection, she received antibiotic injections for several days.

After returning home, Jean found she was more tired than she had expected. With visitors constantly in and out, Jean had little time to be alone with the baby and her older son. Also, the headaches that had developed in the hospital persisted for 10 weeks and greatly affected Jean's recovery at home.

She had some help from the health visitor and community nurses, which was much appreciated. A baby-carrier was devised to enable her to carry her baby and push her wheelchair at the same time. To avoid getting up at night, nappy-changing supplies, a bottle of formula milk on ice, and a bottle-warmer were left beside her bed. Before long, Jean felt things were back to normal.

(From a paper presented to the 1981 Annual National Symposium on Sexuality and Disability by Wilma Asrael, Mary Bolding, and Paula Eckard, reproduced with the kind permission of the authors.)

Contacts

The spinal unit or orthopaedic hospital where you were originally treated is likely to be your main source of medical attention and advice and you can ask to be put in touch with other young mothers from there.

Spinal Injuries Association
76 St James's Lane
London W1
Tel. 081-444 2121

Runs a link scheme that can also put you in touch with other mothers.

References

Asrael, W., Bolding, M., and Eckard, P. (1981) 'Childbirth preparation for the pregnant quadriplegic woman', *Childbirth Educator*.

*Miller, J. B. (May 1982) *Obstetrical Management of the Spinal-Cord-Injured Patient*. Available from Catawba Women's Center, Hickory, North Carolina, USA.

* Verduyn, W. H. (October 1983) 'Spinal cord injured women, pregnancy and delivery'. A patient survey and literature review.

Winkelaar, E. (1986) 'Pregnancy and spinal cord injury', *Rehabilitation Gazette* 27(2).

(* Publications that may prove difficult for readers without a medical education to follow.)

Further reading

Mooney, T. O., Cole, T. M., and Chilgren, R. A. (1975) *Sexual Options for Paraplegics and Quadriplegics*, Little, Brown and Co.
A lot of informative and reassuring discussion of all aspects of sexual awareness and communication accompanied by photographs.

Morris, J. (ed.) (1989) *Able Lives: women's experience of paralysis*, The Women's Press.
This makes excellent reading and has a chapter on pregnancy and motherhood.

Nass, A. (December 1986) 'Spinal cord-injured women: pregnancy and delivery', *Paraplegia News*, Paralysed Veterans of America.

Oliver, M. J., Zarb, G., Silver, J., Moore, M., and Salisbury, V. (1989) *Walking into Darkness – The Experience of Spinal Cord Injury*, Macmillan.

Taggie, J. M. and Manley, M. S. (1979) *A Handbook on Sexuality after Spinal Cord Injury*, Englewood, Colorado: Craig Hospital.

The Spinal Injuries Association now keep a collection of accounts of motherhood by women with spinal cord injuries, all of which make interesting and enlightening reading.

The medical library at Stoke Mandeville Hospital in Aylesbury, Bucks, keeps a comprehensive bibliography of books and journal articles dealing with paraplegia and all aspects of sexual function in men and women. Most of these are specialist texts but would make useful reading for any interested doctor or paramedic.

Chapter nineteen

Visual impairment

This book should be available on cassette, but I include this chapter for the benefit of professional carers and relatives who can pass on the information to a woman with a visual impairment.

What is visual impairment?

Visual impairment ranges from complete loss of sight to partial sight and this means the person has difficulty seeing things clearly or at all. Only 10 per cent of the visually impaired can see nothing at all. There are many different sorts of visual impairment: a person may have no central vision but have peripheral vision or, alternatively, have no peripheral vision and only tunnel vision. Others may see the world as through cracked glass. Still others may be able to see high colour contrasts.

Who gets it ?

In Britain, the Royal National Institute for the Blind (RNIB) estimate that there are 300,000 people with severe visual handicap and about 82,000 who are partially sighted. There may be many more who do not register as blind.

How does it affect daily life?

The main problems are obviously in reading and getting around, but other day-to-day problems may be less obvious – not being able to see expressions on people's faces, not being able to choose products in shops without assistance.

What is the cause?

There are many different causes for visual impairment. These include accidents, childhood illnesses (such as meningitis), diabetes and, very rarely, genetic causes such as retinitis pigmentosa, congenital cataracts or albinism. Some eye conditions are degenerative.

Can it be cured?

This depends on the cause. If deterioration of sight is due to an illness, this can sometimes be arrested. Some conditions can be operated on with varying degrees of success.

Can a woman with a visual impairment have children?

Yes, there are no reproductive problems associated with blindness, only practical ones. Many, many women with visual handicaps have successfully raised children.

Will it affect fertility?

No.

What is the risk to the baby?

For the few genetically related eye conditions, there is obviously a risk that you will pass the condition on to the child, so you should seek genetic counselling to ascertain this before deciding whether to go ahead. Otherwise the only risk is to do with the practical problems of looking after the baby.

How will the pregnancy affect the visual impairment?

There are very few eye conditions that will be affected by pregnancy. One such is if the impairment was caused by treatment for a tumour, in which case the high blood pressure sometimes associated with pregnancy may cause problems.

There is one symptom of pregnancy which may cause more problems for visually impaired women. This is the swelling of the fingers that sometimes occurs towards the end of the pregnancy. It obviously affects the sensitivity with which you can feel things when touching. It is annoying but should pass shortly after your baby is born.

Special care during pregnancy

The only special care is to be even more vigilant about avoiding falls as the growing baby will no doubt change your centre of gravity.

In hospital

Ask someone to orient you so that you are familiar with the layout of, for example, the labour ward, delivery suite, special care unit, postnatal ward, and bathrooms. A bed or room near a bathroom should be requested, and you should resist attempts to move you around once you are settled in. During labour your partner can be your guide to who is coming in and out and what they are doing, or a sympathetic midwife can help with this, perhaps with a little prompting.

On the postnatal ward, if you are in a room to yourself, one blind mother suggested putting up a note on the door asking people to announce themselves when entering or leaving the room. This avoids the anxiety of not knowing who is in the room and what they are up to, and also the embarrassment of being left talking into thin air.

If you have a guide dog you will need to discuss whether he can stay with you in hospital. Talk to the midwifery manager at the hospital about this.

Breastfeeding

Breastfeeding is far preferable to bottle-feeding as the sterilising and making up of formula milk is fiddly and time-consuming if you have a visual impairment. Breastfeeding enables more closeness with the baby – you can feel the facial muscles smiling and respond to the baby more immediately with your own smiles. Get the midwife to check that you don't have inverted nipples or any other problems that might stop you breastfeeding successfully.

Can my child see?

This is often a worry, even for mothers whose visual handicap is not genetic. A visit from an eye specialist soon after the birth should be arranged to give peace of mind.

Looking after baby

Since this is likely to be the major challenge, I am including a selection of tips from other blind mothers.

- Get to know neighbours; have a GP and health visitor who are supportive and will pop round any time to check up on wounds, minor illnesses, etc.
- Many tasks are easier performed on your lap than on, for example, a nappy-changing table in the early weeks.
- There are many pieces of equipment available for blind mothers – contact the RNIB for more details.
- Storage of baby's things on shelves that are marked with some sort of touch-marker and replaced in the same place each time will make life easier. If you are worried about colour coordination, put matching clothes together or mark with, for example, safety pins or coded buttons available from RNIB shop.
- Hold baby upright against you when moving around house so as to avoid banging her head on jutting out shelves, etc.
- Bath baby with you in big bath or in baby bath in big bath. Always put cold water in first and then hot to avoid scalds.
- Slings for carrying the baby around in the early weeks are more convenient than prams and leave hands free for a cane or guide dog. Later on a back-pack is useful if you are fairly strong!

As the baby gets older . . . .

You will need to be more vigilant about dangers for a mobile baby. A large play-pen from an early age is useful, particularly the lightweight ones which can be moved around the house with you. Avoid overhanging tablecloths and unstable furniture. Put latches on cupboard doors, cover electrical sockets. Don't leave hot drinks around. Never leave your baby loose and alone.

Use harnesses on the baby when crawling and toddling. Older babies should be fed in highchairs in the kitchen or other room with a wipe-clean floor, and should wear the overall type of plastic bib.

A musical potty was highly recommended – also, don't rush to get your baby out of nappies as unseen puddles around the house can be dangerous and unhygienic.

You may need to be prepared to ask for help with the following aspects of parenting, particularly if your husband also has a visual handicap:

- Pushing prams
- Dealing with wounds
- Outings to new places
- Reading and writing
- Swimming

If you decide to have more than one child it is probably best to wait until the first is old enough to be fairly independent before embarking on another.

Visual impairment: case history 1

I was 31, married, and working as an audiotypist in Reading when I began to think about having children. I am partially sighted as a result of oxygen deficiency at a premature birth. My husband is also partially sighted though his condition was not diagnosed or treated until he was 9 years old and the cause is still not known.

We consulted our eye specialist about the possibility of our child being partially sighted. He investigated my medical history and said there were unlikely to be any problems with the child's sight. So we went ahead and I conceived straight away.

As I knew little about pregnancy and childbirth, I read everything I could get my hands on and found most things useful to some degree. The tapes from Hethersett College were not crucial to me as I can read print but I recommend them for those who can't.

I had no particular problems through my pregnancy except that I was very tired throughout (due to a very demanding job) and had bouts of backache (probably more from bending over a VDU for hours than from the pregnancy!).

Towards the end of the pregnancy my blood pressure shot up so I was admitted to hospital for a few days and then sent home to rest until the baby arrived.

I attended antenatal classes at the GP surgery but found them difficult to follow, particularly the exercises. The teachers did try to help but as there were 16 in the class it wasn't always easy.

Lots of the classes were taken up with exercises and breathing but I had little enthusiasm for them when I was back home. I felt that the classes were intended to help with the birth and looking after the baby rather than yourself.

The midwife came to our home and made sure I had everything for the birth and the health visitor also introduced herself beforehand. I consider them both to have been an excellent help – they also checked that forms were filled in at right times for maternity grants, etc.

On the day of labour I went in right at the start and it was 16 hours before our daughter was born.

I felt fairly well looked after in labour. The doctors were a bit cool but I thought the midwives were great. My only criticism is that during the second stage when I needed them most they were busy doing paperwork because it was a change of shift, and also some of the monitoring equipment didn't work properly so more attention was lavished on that.

Our baby was given to me straightaway and I put her to the breast. My feelings at the time, I remember, were: very tired, not very thrilled with life, and in great pain from bruising of the ribs caused by the baby kicking during labour.

Our eye specialist came to see our daughter within 24 hours of her birth and declared her eyes well. He saw her again at 3 months and annually since – her sight is near-perfect.

I spent a week in hospital which I didn't enjoy much. I found it confusing because I had been on one side of the corridor before the birth and then, disorientated, on the other side afterwards. I never did work out where I was, so used the same loo and bathroom all the time – I didn't have a shower. I was moved to a smaller unit after 48 hours which I hated because it was so quiet! Also, it was extremely hot summer weather and I found it difficult to stay comfortable.

Breastfeeding and learning babycare were hard but not impossible, and back home my husband had taken 3 weeks off work to help. I refused a home help when offered one as I did not really feel I needed one with the first child. Some of the advice I would give is as follows:

- *Get to know your neighbours before pregnancy.*
- *Get to know about local facilities for new mothers.*
- *Get a GP who is willing to visit any time – and make sure his surgery is as near as possible. I didn't and had to change later on, which was a blow to us all.*

- *Avoid bottle-feeding if you possibly can!*
- *Have a dimmer switch in the nursery and keep it low all the time so you can see where you are going immediately.*
- *Don't buy a crib – use a drawer and put it inside the cot – saves tripping over those dreadful fragile legs.*
- *Buy plenty of harnesses so you have one on each highchair, pram, etc., plus a set of reins. Saves fighting to get them on and off all the time.*
- *Later on, feed at all times in the kitchen, on a wipe-clean floor, and use the overall-type bibs. Little bibs are useless for the partially sighted as the baby knocks the food around to places you can't always spot.*

My daughter is now 4 years old and seems well-adjusted to our visual handicaps. We have not yet made any attempt to explain them specifically. She understands that, for example, Daddy can't read to her before 10 am (because his eyes take time to start focussing in the morning). My hand–eye coordination isn't great, so her drawing is better than mine. But there have been no major problems.

My sight is slowly deteriorating and I have now got stronger lenses to be able to read small-print, but I think this is just due to age.

We decided before Hazel was born that we would have just one child and have kept to that. This is not particularly because of our visual handicaps, just a personal choice.

Visual impairment: case history 2

I am blind (due to my mother's contact with rubella during pregnancy) and my husband is also blind (due to oxygen tent treatment as a premature baby). I received genetic counselling while still at school and my husband also knew that his condition was not likely to be passed on. So our worries were not so much about the pregnancy as how we would cope with a child. I read some material produced by the NCT Health Education council and a few leaflets specifically for blind mothers. The material available in Braille and on tape then (1985) was not very detailed and needs updating as there are very many additional services, groups, and products now available which could help blind parents with young children.

On the whole I was well looked after in my first pregnancy. My GP was not particularly supportive but I found the antenatal clinic staff at the hospital very friendly and encouraging. I attended parentcraft classes at the hospital and the Sister there was very keen to help us. She made a tape for me of the exercises so that I could become familiar with them before the classes started. I was also allowed to examine any models befor a class started and films were described as necessary.

I received no specific advice from the health visitor about equipment specific to my disability but I had a supportive family who had a lot of ideas.

On the big day I went into hospital about 5 hours after contractions had started and it was another 8 before the baby was born. I had a normal delivery which was only really painful for the last 3 hours. I had pethidine and asked for gas-and-oxygen, though my husband could tell from the sound I made that I wasn't using it properly. I walked around for as long as possible, but once on the bed, was put on the monitor, which I found restricting.

I had to have an episiotomy, which I found the most painful experience of all. I was generally too taken up with the labour to be very aware of how it was managed in the second stage, though in the first everyone had been very kind. My husband was more aware of the little things he was not happy with, but, by and large, he enjoyed the experience.

I held my daughter straightaway but only for a moment. I asked to put her to the breast but she was whisked away to have the mucus sucked out that she had swallowed during birth. I felt disappointed as I was afraid she would not be so keen to suck later on, relieved that the pain had stopped, but other than that I didn't feel much for a while.

On the postnatal ward I managed fairly well. In general, I could get around, but one big irritation was that the shower and bidet nearest us were out of order so that, by the end of the week, when I had learnt to manage the baby alone, I was still having to summon help for myself as the route to the other shower on the ward was too complicated to memorise in the time. As for help with breastfeeding and babycare, I felt very well served on the whole. Occasionally, I was muddled by conflicting advice from the staff. At first I had to summon someone to help me get the baby latched on to the breast but they never minded this. I was given a choice of whether I had my own room or went in with the other mums – I chose the latter, which meant I realised others had the same problems as myself. The matron asked the staff not to help me unless I asked for it and told me she had done so. Some staff did change nappies without being asked but I was quite glad of this as I found there were a lot of new things to learn all at once.

I had problems learning to handle the baby in that all the tasks were unfamiliar and also, for the first few days, I could not really rely on my sense of touch as the swelling in my fingers towards the end of pregnancy did not go down straight away.

I was given some help with all these tasks but did not really feel happy until I had found my own routines with them at home. I was helped with bathing the baby three times during the week I was in hospital, and this I found very helpful. I immediately felt happy with it when I first tried it alone.

I went home when the baby was a week old and found the day-to-day care much easier at home as I was beginning to feel I knew her and I could arrange things to suit me rather than doing it in the confined space of my part of the room in hospital. My husband had taken 2 weeks off work and my mum also stayed with us for the first 3 days and came over when she could after that.

Looking back, I can't honestly think of anything I would have done differently, though I think we are particularly lucky in having a model baby, very supportive friends and family, and understanding health professionals. At no time did anyone imply that we should not, as a blind couple, have children. Our daughter has perfect sight.

I would advise first-time mothers with a visual handicap to talk to any visually handicapped mums they know, or to take steps to get to know some, as I have found the advice of other blind mothers invaluable. Also get to know many sighted parents and children through the NCT, etc., and to find out about local facilities and national organisations, for the blind as well as for all.

I have also found that I am much happier now that I have learnt not to try to be fiercely independent, in other words, I take up many more offers of help, and even ask for it – something I very rarely did before I had a child to think of as well as myself. It's difficult to advise others about this, however, as it is so dependent on temperament, but I have found it is the only way I find time to do many of the things I need or want to do.

Contacts

Advice for blind parents run by:

Mr and Mrs R. Hinds
Tel. 0732 61803

Royal National Institute for the Blind
24-hour advice line 0732 61477

Partially Sighted Society
206 Great Portland St
London W1N 6AA
Tel. 071-387 8840

British Retinitis Pigmentosa Society
Mrs L. M. Drummond Walker
24 Palmer Close
Redhill
Surrey RH1 4BX
Tel. 0737-61937

Torch Trust for the Blind
Torch House
Hallaton
Market Harborough
Leicestershire
Tel. 085889 301

This is a Christian organisation that provides fellowship and support through a nationwide network of groups.

There are also a number of blind mother and baby groups springing up around the country: contact the NCT Contact Register (Tel. 081-992 8637) if you want to know whether there is one local to you or if you are planning to start one.

Local talking newspapers are a good way of finding other blind mothers with young children in your area.

References and further reading
(most available in Braille or on cassette)

A variety of information on pregnancy and childcare for blind mothers is available from:

Yvonne Rowe
Hethersett College (RNIB)
32 Gatton Road
Wray Common
Reigate
Surrey RH2 0HD
Tel. 07372-45555

A guide for midwives and health visitors is also available from the same address.

The RNIB also has a publication for hospital staff: RNIB (1987) *Helping Visually Handicapped People in Hospital.*

There is a chapter on visual impairment in:

Bullard, D.G. and Knight, S.E. (eds) *Sexuality and Physical Disability – Personal Perspectives*, Mosby.

The following American article is not available on cassette or in Braille as far as I know, but makes interesting reading as it follows the experiences of ten blind mothers as they coped with the problems of caring for young children:

Ware, M. A. and Schwab, L. O. (1971) 'The blind mother providing care for an infant', *The New Outlook for the Blind* 65:169–73.

For antenatal teachers:

Bobek, B. (1984) 'Use the common senses: childbirth education for blind and visually impaired persons', *Journal of Visual Impairment and Blindness*, pp. 350–1.

General reading:

(1970) 'Hints for blind mothers', *The New Beacon: The Journal of Blind Welfare* 65:58–63.

Some helpful organisations

AIMS
The Association for Improvements in the Maternity Services
40 Kingswood Road
London NW6
Tel. 071-278 5628

Offers information and advice on all aspects of maternity care, including parents' rights, the choices available, etc.

DIAL UK
National Association of Disablement Information and Advice Services
Victoria Buildings
117 High Street
Clay Cross
Chesterfield
Derbyshire S45 9DZ
Tel. 0246 864498

They can give you the number of your local DIAL (Disablement Information and Advice Line) which is run by disabled people to provide information and advice on local services, etc.

Disabled Living Foundation
380–384 Harrow Road
London W9 2HU
Tel. 071-289 6111

Provides a specialist advisory service on aids and equipment.

Homestart Consultancy
140 New Walk
Leicester LE1 7JL
Tel. 0533 554988

Local Homestart schemes now exist in many parts of the UK to provide support, friendship and practical help to parents of under-fives.

Independent Living Fund
PO Box 183
Nottingham NG8 3RD

May provide grants for those who are on attendance allowance towards childcare costs.

Mary Marlborough Lodge
Nuffield Orthopaedic Centre
Headington
Oxford OX3 7LD
Tel. 0865 64811

A residential assessment centre to help disabled parents adjust to life with a new baby.

Maternity Alliance
15 Britannia Street
London WC1X 9JP
Tel. 071-837 1266

As its name suggests, this has member groups which cover every aspect of pregnancy and motherhood. It campaigns for better services for parents and babies. In particular, they can advise on financial benefits available to mothers. In 1989 they set up a Disability Working Group.

National Council for One Parent Families
255 Kentish Town Road
London NW5 2LX
Tel. 071-267 1361

Provides free and confidential advice on all aspects of single parenting.

NCT
National Childbirth Trust
Alexandra House
Oldham Terrace
Acton
London W3 6NH
Tel. 081-992 8637

Provides a great variety of free pamphlets on breastfeeding. Can also tell you where your local branch is situated. This provides antenatal and postnatal support activities.

OPUS
Organisation for Parents under Stress
106 Godstone Road
Whyteleafe
CR3 0EB
Tel. 081-645 0469

Will put you in touch with a local helpline.

REMAP
25 Mortimer St
London W1N 8AB
Tel. 081-637 5400

Provides volunteers with technical expertise to design and make items of equipment to meet the specific needs of individuals with a disability.

Stillbirth and Neonatal Death Society
28 Portland Place
London W1N 3DE
Tel. 071-436 5881

Working Mothers' Association
23 Webbs Road
London SW11 6RU
Tel. 071-228 3757

Self-help organisation for working parents. It has a network of local groups to provide an informal support system for working mothers.

Bibliography on the effect of parental physical disability on children

Buck, F. M. and Hohmann, G. W. (1979) 'Parenthood in spinal cord injured fathers: an investigation of their adult children', *Paraplegia News*, pp. 30–2.

Buck, F. M. and Hohmann, G. W. (1983) 'Parental disability and children's adjustment', *Annual Review of Rehabilitation* 3, New York: Springer Publishing Company.

Collis, G. M. and Bryant, C. A. (1981) 'Interactions between blind parents and their young children', *Child Care Health and Development* 7:41–50.

DiCarprio, N. S. (1971) 'Factors affecting the child's evaluation of the visually handicapped parent', *The New Outlook for the Blind* 65:181–3.

Frankenburg, F. R., Sloman, L., and Perry, A. (1985) 'Issues in the therapy of hearing children with deaf parents', *Canadian Journal of Psychiatry* 30:98–102.

Hallie (1978) 'Psychodynamic conflicts in hearing children of deaf parents', *International Journal of Psychoanalysis and Psychotherapy* 7:305–15.

Kirshbaum, M. (1988) 'Parents with physical disabilities and their babies', *Zero to Three* 23(11):509–12.

Meadow, K. P., Greenberg, M. T., and Erting, C. (1983) 'Attachment behaviour of deaf children with deaf parents', *Journal of the American Academy of Child Psychiatry* 22:23–8.

Thurman, S. K. (1985) *Children of Handicapped Parents, Research and Clinical Perspectives*, London: Academic Press.

Vash, C. (1983) *The Psychology of Disability*, New York: Springer Publishing. See chapter on the family.

Weiner, C. L. (1984) 'The Burden of Rheumatoid Arthritis', in *Chronic Illness and the Quality of Life*, Strauss, A. L. (ed.), St Louis: C. V. Mosby, pp. 88–98.

Selection of contacts and references for disabling conditions not covered in Part 2

Most of the self-help groups listed here can put you in touch with other mothers.

AIDS

AIDS and Childbirth, free leaflet produced by AVERT

AVERT (AIDS Education and Research Trust)
PO Box 91
Horsham
West Sussex RH13 7YR

Brittle bones

Mason, M. (January 1986) 'Women, disability and reproductive rights', *GLC Women's Committee Bulletin*. Micheline Mason has brittle bones.

Brittle Bone Society
Unit 4 Block 20
Carlunie Road
Dunsinane Industrial Estate
Dundee DD2 3QT
Tel. 0382 817771

The Brittle Bone Society can help put you in touch with other women with the disorder.

Cancer

Allen, H. U. and Nisker, G. A. (eds) (1986) *Cancer and Pregnancy – Therapeutic Guidelines*, New York: Futura.

British Association of Cancer United Patients
121–123 Charterhouse Street
London EC1M 6AA
Tel. 071-608 1661

BACUP provides individual counselling and hopes to produce some written information on cancer and pregnancy in the near future.

Cystic fibrosis

Barby, T. and Bobrow, M. *Genetics and Tests During Pregnancy*, and

Walters, S. and Hodson, M. *Fertility, Pregnancy and Contraception in Cystic Fibrosis*, are both comprehensive, authoritative booklets available free from:

Cystic Fibrosis Research Trust/Association of CF Adults
Alexandra House
5 Blyth Road
Bromley, Kent BR1 3RS
Tel. 081-464 7211

Friedreich's and Cerebellar Ataxia

Friedreich's & Cerebellar Ataxia Group
Burleigh Lodge
Knowle Lane
Cranleigh GU6 8RD
Tel. 0483 272741

Inflammatory bowel disease

Mayberry, J. F. (1988) 'Assessment of an information booklet on pregnancy for patients with inflammatory bowel disease', *Journal of Obstetrics and Gynaecology* 9:14–17.

Kidney disease

Davison, J. M. (1987) 'Pregnancy and motherhood following renal trans-
plantation', *Midwifery* 3:125–32.

Mrs Elizabeth Ward also provides advice and counselling at

The British Kidney Patient Association
Bordon
Hants
Tel. 04203 2021/2

Muscular dystrophy

Muscular Dystrophy Group of Great Britain and Northern Ireland
Nattrass House
35 Macaulay Road
London SW4 0QP
Tel. 071-720 8055

Myalgic encephalomyelitis

ME Association
Mrs P. Searles
The Moss
Third Avenue
Stanford-le-Hope
Essex SS17 8EL
Tel. 0375 642466

The ME Association produces a free leaflet entitled 'Pregnancy and
Myalgic Encephalomyelitis' with information and advice.

Myasthenia gravis

British Association of Myasthenics
Keynes House
77 Nottingham Road
Derby DE1 3QS
Tel. 0332 290219

Parkinson's disease

Young Alert Parkinsons, Partners and Relatives
(YAPP&RS)
c/o Paul and Diana Lewin
31 Kilmahew Avenue
Cardross
Dumbarton G82 5NG
Tel. 0389 841763

Polio

British Polio Fellowship
Bell Close
West End Road
Ruislip
Middlesex HA4 6LP
Tel. 0895 675515

Sickle cell

The Sickle Cell Society
Green Lodge
Barretts Green Road
London NW10 7AP
Tel. 081-961 7795

The Sickle Cell Society now has a telephone counsellor at the London office whom you can call for information and advice if you do not live near to one of the ten national sickle cell centres.

Systemic lupus erythematosis

British SLE Aid Group
25 Linden Crescent
Woodford Green
Essex OG8 1DG

The Lupus Society
5 Grosvenor Crescent
London SW1X 7ER
Tel. 071-235 0902

Thalassaemia

UK Thalassaemia Society
107 Nightingale Road
London N8 7QY
Tel. 081-348 0437

Thalidomide

Kpakiwa, R. (1987) 'Janette, a special mother (thalidomide)', *Nursing Times* 83(49):41–3.

Chamberlain, G. (1989) 'The obstetric problems of the thalidomide children', *British Medical Journal* 298:6.

Appendix D

Contacts outside Britain

Most of the professional and disability organisations listed in this book that exist in Britain have equivalents in other countries. If you are unfamiliar with the ones that could provide support relevant to your needs, a good starting point is to contact your national disability organisations as listed in the telephone directories. These keep information relating to most aspects of disability and can therefore usually help put you in touch with local organisations and sources of support.

A few examples are given below:

Australia

Australian Council for the Rehabilitation of the Disabled
33 Thesiger Court
Deakin
ACT 2600
Tel. (62) 824 333

Can provide information relating to all disability organisations and self-help groups throughout Australia.

Nursing Mothers' Association of Australia
National Headquarters
5 Glendale Street
Nunawading
Victoria 3131
Tel. (03) 877 5011

Canada

Canada Rehabilitation Council for the Disabled
Suite 2110, One Yonge Street
Toronto
Ontario
M5E 1E5
Tel. (416) 862 0340

Can provide details of national disability organisations, self-help groups and services for people with disabilities.

Tali Conine
School of Rehabilitation Medicine
University of British Columbia
Vancouver
British Columbia
V6T 1W5

Contact for Parenting and Disability annotated bibliography and also a guide to aids and adaptations for disabled parents.

New Zealand

Disabled Persons Assembly (New Zealand) Inc.
PO Box 27-186
67 Hanky Street
Wellington
Tel. (04) 857 828

Can provide information about most disability organisations and self-help groups operating in New Zealand.

USA

There are a large number of national and local organisations that can help provide information, counselling and support to people with disabilities embarking on parenthood. The following list is not comprehensive but should help get you started.

American Association of Psychoprophylaxis in Obstetrics
1411 K St. N.W.
Washington, DC 20005

ASPO/Lamaze (Childbirth organisation)
1840 Wilson Boulevard
Arlington
Virginia 22201

Childbirth Without Pain Education Association
1840 Wilson Boulevard
Arlington
Virginia 22201

Coalition on Sexuality and Disability
841 Broadway, Suite 205
New York
NY 10003
Tel. (212) 242 3900

Disability International USA
c/o The Paralysed Veterans of America
801 18th St NW
Washington, DC 20006
Tel. (202) 872 1300

This acts as a clearing house for information about disability organisations and self-help groups throughout the USA. *Paraplegia News*, a monthly newsletter, is published by this organisation.

Information Center for Individuals with Disabilities (ICID)
20 Park Plaza Rm 330
Boston MA 02116
Tel. (617) 727 5540

An organisation that seeks to assist individuals with disabilities in learning about the appropriate resources, agencies and facts that promote a more independent lifestyle.

International Childbirth Education Association
PO Box 20048
Minneapolis MN 55420
Tel. (616) 854 8660

National Rehabilitation Association
633 S. Washington Street
Alexandria
Virginia 22314
Tel. (703) 836 0850

National Rehabilitation Information Centre (NARIC)
8455 Coleville Road, Suite 935
Silver Spring
Maryland 20910-3319

National Rehabilitation Information Center (NARIC)
4407 Eighth Street, N.E.
Washington, DC 20017
Tel. (202) 635 5826

A major source of information on all aspects of disability.

The Paralysed Veterans of America
(publish *Paraplegia News*)
5201 N. 19th Ave, Suite 111
Phoenix
Arizona 85015–9986

Sexuality and Disability Training Center
University Hospital
75 East Newton Street
Boston MA 02118
Tel. (617) 247 5291

A regional centre providing psychological, medical and educational services to people with physical disabilities and other interested persons.

Through The Looking Glass
801 Peralta Avenue
Berkeley
California 94707

A recently established organisation for parents with disabilities. It publishes a regular newsletter.

The last word. . . .

If you think you can cope, go ahead and don't be put off by people who say 'she will never cope with a baby' but who, a year later, say 'Haven't you done well?' It is hard work and very, very tiring, but the rewards are numerous.

Mother with arthritis

Is it worth it? What would any other parent say? I am a parent first and disabled second. We have our problems but so does every other family. We're not so different.

Mother with polio

I have been paralysed for 29 years since a road accident but despite being a paraplegic delivered three healthy sons who are now in their twenties. We all enjoy each other's company and have never had any serious problems because of my disability – my sons are happy, intelligent and out-going and have never been anything other than proud of their mother.

Paraplegic mother

I survive by not blaming my disability when I have a problem. My children have learned to do the same.

Mother with arthritis

Index